950

COLOUR
Sports Medicine

Eugene Sherry MB ChB, MPH, MD, (Orth)
Senior Lecturer in Orthopaedic Surgery,
University of Sydney

Consultant Orthopaedic Surgeon,
Nepean Hospital, Penrith
Jamison Private Hospital, Sydney
Hills Private Hospital, Sydney
Sydney Adventist Hospital, Sydney

D1369184

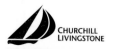

CHURCHILL
LIVINGSTONE

EDINBURGH LONDON MADRID MELBOURNE NEW YORK AND TOKYO 1997

CHURCHILL LIVINGSTONE
Medical Division of Pearson Professional Limited

Distributed in the United States of America by
Churchill Livingstone Inc., 650 Avenue of the Americas,
New York, N.Y. 10011, and by associated companies,
branches and representatives throughout the world.

© Pearson Professional Limited 1997

First published 1997

ISBN 0-443-05482-7

British Library Cataloguing in Publication Data
A catalogue record for this book is available from the British
Library.

Library of Congress Cataloging in Publication Data
A catalog record for this book is available from the Library of
Congress.

Medical knowledge is constantly changing. As new
information becomes available, changes in treatment,
procedures, equipment and the use of drugs become
necessary. The author and the publishers have, as far as it is
possible, taken care to ensure that the information given in
this text is accurate and up to date. However, readers are
strongly advised to confirm that the information, especially
with regard to drug usage, complies with current legislation
and standards of practice.

Publisher
Michael Parkinson

Project Editor
Barbara Simmons

Project Controller
Kay Hunston

Design Director
Erik Bigland

Produced by Longman Asia Ltd, Hong Kong
SWT/01

Preface

Sports medicine is a new and evolving medical discipline charged with the care of the injured and sick athlete. This text will be useful to medical students, residents, registrars, sports medicine specialists, orthopaedic surgeons, physiotherapists, nurses, coaches and trainers. It will equip the reader with a 'state of the art' knowledge of sports medicine. It is written in a practical style with colour illustrations to highlight the essential and useful topics in this area. For the compilation of the material in this book I have drawn from the experience gained in the management of over 25 000 sporting injuries.

I would like to thank Dr Q. Reeves (Radiologist, Sydney) for contributing radiological material, Margaret Kenny (Jada Art, Sydney) for illustrations and layout, Dr A. Henderson (Intern, Sydney) and Jamison Private Hospital (Penrith, Sydney) for assistance. The following experts wrote chapters:

Dr R. J. Bazina (Intern, Sydney): The Female Athlete
Dr J. E. C. Bentivoglio (Orthopaedic Surgeon, Sydney): Injuries of the Spine
Dr D. J. Bokor (Orthopaedic Surgeon, Sydney): Injuries of the Shoulder, Injuries of the Elbow
Dr W. K. Chung (Orthopaedic Surgeon, Sydney): The Child Athlete
Dr D. B. Kuah (Sports Medicine Specialist, Sydney): Sport and the Environment
Dr J. E. Ireland (Orthopaedic Surgeon, Sydney): Injuries of the Hip and Thigh
Dr V. J. Mamo (Orthopaedic Registrar, Sydney): The Older Athlete
Dr D. C. Yee (Hand Surgeon, Sydney): Injuries of the Hand and Wrist

Sydney, 1996

E.S.

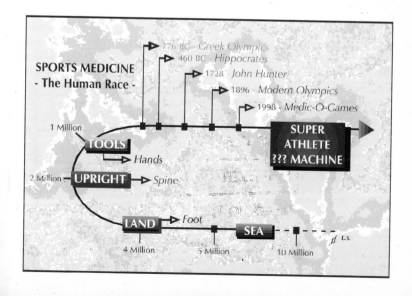

Acknowledgements

Fig. 4: Courtesy of the Australian Picture Library/Allsports Photography USA

Figs 5, 7, 8, 9, 27*, 28†: Courtesy of the Australian Picture Library

Figs 10, 11, 12, 13: Courtesy of LCDR Kevin Boundy, Royal Australian Navy

Fig. 21: Courtesy of John Fairfax and Sons Limited

Fig. 32: Courtesy of Dr J. French

Fig. 171: Courtesy of Allsports USA

*Fleur McIntyre from Australia
†Bin Lu from China

Contents

1. Basic sports science — 1
2. Sport and the environment — 5
3. Sudden death in sport — 15
4. Other significant medical concerns — 21
5. The female athlete — 23
6. Injuries of the shoulder — 31
7. Injuries of the elbow — 41
8. Injuries of the hand and wrist — 49
9. Injuries of the hip, thigh and pelvis — 59
10. Injuries of the knee — 71
11. Injuries of the foot, ankle and leg — 79
12. Injuries of the spine — 91
13. The child athlete — 103
14. The older athlete — 115

Index — 119

1 / Basic sports science

Exercise

Metabolism **Anaerobic metabolism.** This allows for intense and brief periods of exercise (100-m sprint, speed skating). Lactic acid accumulates and limits the duration of exercise (fatigue). Anaerobic muscle fibres are white, fast twitch (type II).

Aerobic metabolism. This uses oxygen and provides for endurance events. It uses red, slow twitch (type I) muscle forces. The relative proportion of type I/II is genetically determined (endurance athletes = type I; sprinters = type II).

Muscle action This follows the *tension/length* curve shown in Figure 1. Concentric contraction causes muscle shortening; eccentric contraction causes lengthening (dampens joint reactive forces).

Training
- *Endurance training* is repetitive and increases the size/efficiency of type I fibres.
- *Sprint training* concentrates on tension development and so selective hypertrophy of type II fibres.

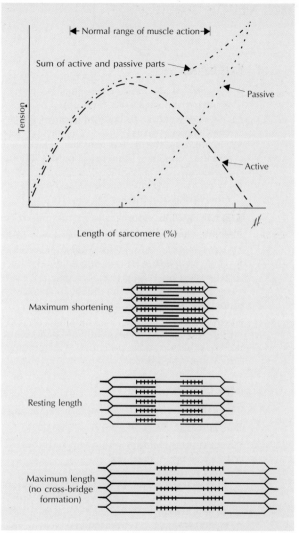

Fig. 1 Tension is dependent upon muscle (sarcomere) length.

Types of exercise

Exercise can be:

- *Isometric*—where tension develops but muscle length is unchanged (against a fixed object).
- *Isotonic*—where muscle moves against a fixed resistance.
- *Isokinetic*—performed at constant velocity with variable resistance (may cause patellofemoral problems).
- *Functional*—dynamic exercises and allows rapid rehabilitation (jump ropes).

Stretching. This improves isometric muscle function, prevents injury and enhances performance (Fig. 2).

Exercise capacity

Cardiovascular function. Maximum exercise capacity is significantly determined by increased O_2 delivery from increased stroke volume/cardiac output, vasodilation and to a lesser extent by increased mitochondrial volume (Fig. 3).

Pulmonary function. The pulmonary system may well determine the limits of athletic performance (the athlete's full metabolic potential). Champions will need large 'vital capacities'.

Sports psychology

This looks at factors determining participation and performance. Areas include:

- motivation (children who compete to beat others are more likely to 'drop out')
- stress/performance (competition)
- interpersonal relations (coach, athlete, parents)
- exercise psychology (exercise probably promotes mental health)
- mental training (success requires a clear focus with certainty and no fear).

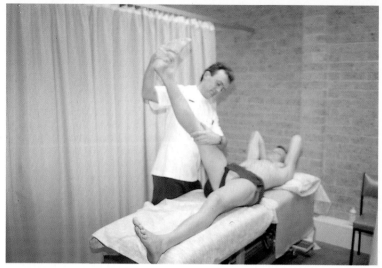

Fig. 2 Close attention to the hamstrings (with stretching) is important to prevent injury and enhance performance.

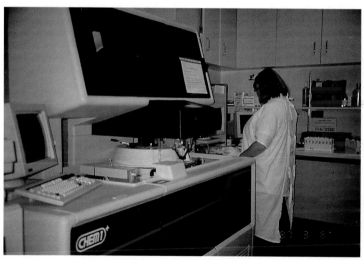

Fig. 3 Performance parameters are tested in the laboratory.

2 / Sport and the environment

Temperature extremes

The human body attempts to maintain its core
temperature (often measured by rectal temperature)
within the normal range of 36.1–37.8°C by a balance
between heat production/gain and heat loss.

Heat illnesses/hyperthermia

Classification Heat illnesses are a spectrum of clinical presentations
classified into mild, moderate or severe (Fig. 4).

Mild: heat fatigue, heat cramps, heat syncope.

Moderate: heat exhaustion.

Severe: heat stroke; >41°C. Reduced level of
consciousness.

Treatment Rest, ice, massage for cramps; rapid cooling (with i.v.
fluids) for severe cases.

Complications These include hypotension, arrhythmias, myocardial
infarct, cardiac failure, convulsions, cerebrovascular
events and coma, gastrointestinal bleeding, liver
damage and renal failure, rhabdomyolysis (breakdown
of skeletal muscle membrane) and disseminated
intravascular coagulation (DIC).

Prevention • Wear appropriate cool, light-coloured clothing.
• Stay well hydrated (Fig. 5).
• Undertake adequate fitness preparation, and heat
  acclimatization if appropriate.
• Avoid exercise in extreme heat (and humidity).

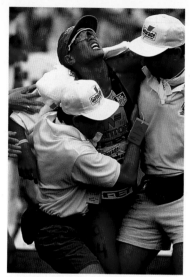

Fig. 4 Heat-affected triathlete.

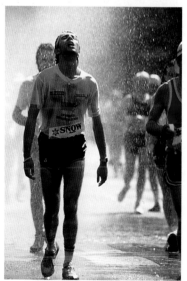

Fig. 5 Water for both hydration and cooling is important in preventing heat illness.

Cold stress/hypothermia

Those at risk of hypothermia include alpine and cross-country skiers, and endurance, adventure and water sports participants.

Classification

Hypothermia can be classified as mild, moderate or severe.

Mild (35–37 °C): cold extremities, shivering, tachycardia, tachypnoea, urinary urgency, slight incoordination.

Moderate (32–34 °C): increased incoordination and clumsiness, reduced shivering, slurred speech, dehydration, fatigue, amnesia, drowsiness, and poor judgement.

Severe (<32 °C): total loss of shivering, inappropriate behaviour, reduced level or loss of consciousness, muscle rigidity, hypotension, pulmonary oedema, extreme bradycardia, and cardiac arrhythmias (especially ventricular fibrillation, VF).

Management

This involves general life-support measures (fluids, nutrition, cardiac support), minimizing further heat loss, and re-warming. Monitor core temperature and vital signs. In severe hypothermia, there must be gentle and minimal handling of the patient for fear of VF arrest. Re-warming may be passive, external active or internal active (controversial topic) (Fig. 6).

Prevention

• Wear appropriate clothing.
• Keep well hydrated and nourished.
• Ensure adequate planning (Fig. 7).
• Achieve appropriate fitness level.
• Avoid exercising to exhaustion.

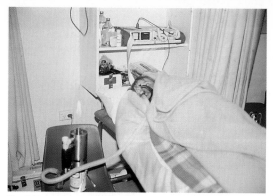

Fig. 6 Treatment for hypothermia (inhalational rewarming)

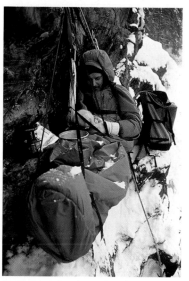

Fig. 7 Good planning and equipment go a long way to prevention of hypothermia.

Altitude medicine

The decrease in barometric pressure and air density which accompanies increases in altitude has both advantages and disadvantages for athletes. Sprinters, are aided by the reduced air resistance whereas endurance athletes are hampered by the lower oxygen concentration (Fig. 8).

Clinical conditions

Mountain sickness. This is usually a temporary condition affecting the first 2 or 3 days of a rapid ascent over 2000 m. Features include headache, dizziness, nausea, vomiting, insomnia, and syncope. Acetazolamide may reduce the symptoms. If the symptoms are severe, return to lower altitudes is indicated.

Altitude cerebral oedema. This is a rare condition which usually occurs on rapid ascents above 4000 m altitude. Symptoms include headache, confusion hallucinations, and reduced level of consciousness or coma. Management involves urgent return to low altitude, oxygen therapy and intravenous corticosteroids.

Altitude pulmonary oedema. This life-threatening condition occurs in the first 3 days of ascent above altitudes of 2000 m and manifests with symptoms of shortness of breath, coughing and copious frothy sputum.

Retinal haemorrhage. Small retinal haemorrhages may occur above altitudes of 4000 m.

Prevention

- Rapid ascents to moderate and high altitudes should be avoided.
- Altitude acclimatization improves pulmonary ventilation, capillarization and increases red blood cell mass and haemoglobin (Fig. 9).
- Awareness and recognition of early symptoms and signs is essential.

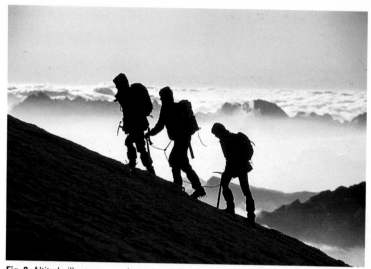

Fig. 8 Altitude illnesses are almost inevitable unless very strict preparation and acclimatization are undertaken.

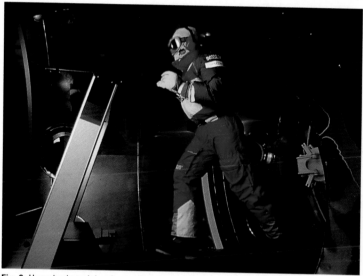

Fig. 9 Hyperbaric training for acclimatization for an attempt on Everest.

Underwater medicine

There are various medical considerations and problems in the popular sport. In underwater diving the most common cause of death is drowning (Fig. 10) whilst the most common problem is decompression sickness. In sea water, pressure increases by one atmosphere with each 10-m increase in depth. Gas-filled spaces undergo their greatest volume changes near the surface. Hence shallow dives may not be safer than deeper dives as is commonly thought.

Decompression sickness (DCS)

DCS involves a wide variety of multi-organ symptoms as a result of the formation of nitrogen bubbles in either the body's tissues or blood during ascent. These symptoms can occur at any time in the first 24 hours following ascent.

Clinical types

Intravascular DCS. Plasma volume is lowered and increased viscosity causes coagulation abnormalities.

Neurological DCS. This involves a wide spectrum of central and peripheral nervous system problems which are due to the increased affinity of nitrogen for myelin.

Cardiorespiratory DCS. Dyspnoea, chest pain and cough ('the chokes') may progress to cardiac arrest if emergency treatment is not instituted.

Musculoskeletal DCS. This is the most common form of DCS and presents as joint pains which may rarely lead to avascular necrosis.

Cutaneous DCS. There is pruritus and a measles-like rash; 'cyanotic marbling' is a sign of severe DCS.

Gastrointestinal DCS. This is associated with abdominal cramps, nausea and anorexia.

Treatment

Early treatment can reverse established symptoms and signs and involves 100% oxygen, intravenous fluids, and the appropriate transport of the patient for recompression (Fig. 11).

CORONER / AUTOPSY
Officially Designated Cause of Death

	ANZ	NUADC
125 causes for 100 victims		
Drowning	86%	74.2%
Pulmonary barotrauma	13%	24.5%
Cardiac	13%	9.1%
Aspiration of vomitus	6%	<1%
Trauma	3%	1.5%
Asthma	2%	
Marine animal injury	1%	
Co - incidental	1%	

Fig. 10 Causes of death in diving accidents.

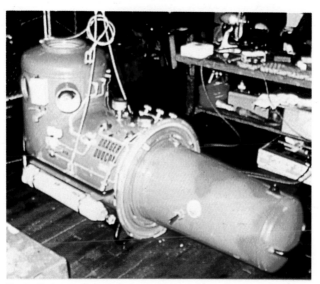

Fig. 11 Early treatment and transport for recompression followed by gradual decompression in a chamber is important in decompression sickness.

Barotrauma (BT)

Barotrauma refers to the injury caused by pressure imbalances between gas spaces in the body and adjacent body tissues or fluids.

Clinical types   ***Middle ear BT.*** This is the most common type of BT with bleeding into the middle ear and tympanic membrane rupture. All cases require audiograms, analgesia and decongestants; antibiotics may also be required.

Inner ear BT. Presents as persisting vertigo and/or tinnitus.

Sinus BT. Presents as blood in the face mask (Fig. 12) and pain, but is not usually serious.

Pulmonary BT. This is the second most common cause of diving deaths and is encountered after rapid or uncontrolled ascent. There may be arterial gas embolism, pneumothorax, surgical emphysema, or pulmonary infarcts. Give 100% oxygen and nurse horizontally if gas embolism is suspected (to avoid air bubbles going to the brain). Stabilize pneumothorax (if present) and recompress.

Prevention of diving accidents

- Pass accredited diving medical.
- Ensure appropriate training certification and safety procedures.
- Current safety equipment should be regularly checked (Fig. 13).

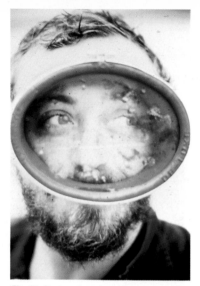

Fig. 12 Ruptured eardrum (barotrauma) in a navy diver.

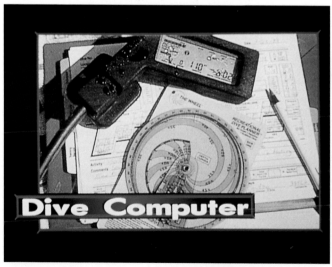

Fig. 13 Current dive equipment is sophisticated and safety orientated.

3 / Sudden death in sport

Sudden and unexpected death is a rare event in sport. In snow skiing one death occurs per every million skier days (1 million skiers on 1 day) (Fig. 14).

Causes The causes are:

- trauma (males <40 years)
- cardiac events (males >40 years)
- hypothermia (children).

Sudden cardiac death

Causes
- In *young athletes* (<35 years) this is usually a myocardial event from an unknown cardiac problem (hypertrophic cardiomyopathy, anomalous coronary arteries, coronary artery disease, conduction system problems).
- In *older athletes* (>35 years) it is usually due to pre-existing coronary artery disease (known in up to 50% of cases). These cases should be preventable.
- In the *old athlete* (>50 years) sudden death is from hyperthermia (hypothermia if in water). There may be a dietary deficiency.

Traumatic deaths

Causes These are due to injuries of:

- the head (Fig. 16)
- the neck (Fig. 15; see also pp. 91–98)
- the chest
- the abdomen.

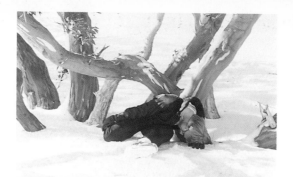

Fig. 14 Sudden death on the slopes (acute subdural haemorrhage; 35-year-old male).

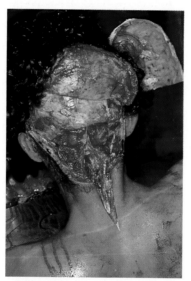

Fig. 15 Cervical crush fracture (C2) in a cross-country (nordic) skier.

Head injuries

Intracranial

These are not uncommon in contact/collision sports (Fig. 16). They can be diffuse or focal.

Diffuse. These may be:

- *mild*—there is no loss of consciousness but a variable period of amnesia
- *classic*—there is definite loss of consciousness
- *diffuse axonal*—loss of consciousness is >6 hours with residual neurological and personality deficiencies.

Focal. These are intracranial haematomas (cerebral contusion, intracerebral extradual/subdural haematomas diagnosed on computerized tomography (CT) of the head; (Fig. 17).

Treatment   Treatment includes resuscitation and surgical evacuation of the haematoma.

Extracranial: faciomaxillary injuries

Extracranial injuries are common in contact and high-speed sports (such as football and skiing). Whilst most are minor, there is a potential for major airways problems and disfigurement. Injuries include fractures of the facial skeleton, facial lacerations and dental injuries (Fig. 18, p. 20). Mouth guards and helmets can prevent such injuries. Fractures may involve the mandible or maxilla (zygoma and orbits) (Fig. 19, p. 20).

Treatment   Treatment includes airways management, control of bleeding (nasal packing; surgical intervention for intracranial bleeding), and surgical stabilization within 3 weeks.

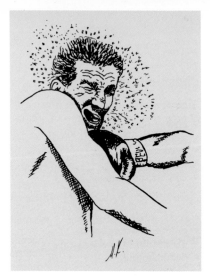

Fig. 16 A right hook in boxing causing the head to spin with damaging torsional and concussional forces applied to the brain.

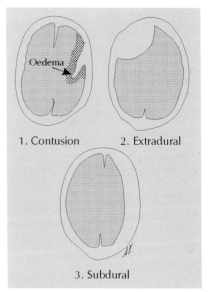

Oedema

1. Contusion   2. Extradural

3. Subdural

Fig. 17 A CT will delineate contusion, extradural haemorrhage and subdural haemorrhage.

Chest injuries

An *immediate* threat to life is caused by:

- airway obstruction
- tension/open pneumothorax
- massive haemothorax
- flail chest
- cardiac tamponade.

Potentially life-threatening problems are:

- myocardial contusion
- pulmonary contusion
- disruption of aorta/airways/oesophagus
- major hernia.

Treatment Accurate diagnosis and resuscitation (with chest tube for pneumothorax) are essential (Fig. 20).

Abdominal injuires

Abdominal injuries are usually the result of blunt trauma in a multi-trauma patient. CT of the abdomen and peritoneal lavage may be necessary.

Resuscitation

Resuscitation involves simultaneous prioritized evaluation and treatment, i.e.:

- *Primary survey*—airways, breathing, circulation
- *Resuscitation*—ventilation, fluids, electrical/support drugs
- *Secondary survey*—for potential problems and need for surgery.

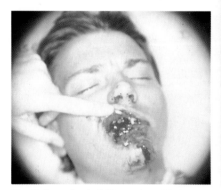

Fig. 18 Extensive facial laceration with dental injuryand broken jaw (skier).

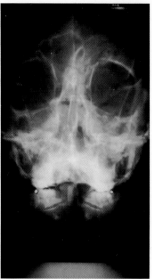

Fig. 19 Cross-country skier with fractured maxilla extending into orbit.

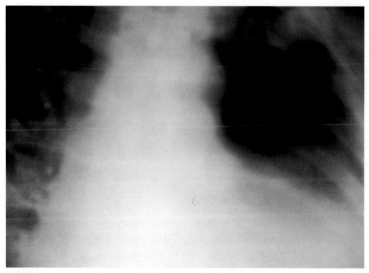

Fig. 20 Pneumothorax from multiple fractured ribs (skier).

4 / Other significant medical concerns

Other medical problems

- Upper respiratory tract infections may (rarely) cause sudden cardiac death (arrhythmia or viral myocarditis).
- Glandular fever may predispose to splenic rupture, myocarditis, or persistent fatigue.
- Hepatatis (resume normal activities when asymptomatic).
- Chronic fatigue syndrome (symptomatic treatment only).
- HIV infection (normal social/sport contact okay).

Disabled athletes
To watch children with physical (diabetes, epilepsy, amputees) and social/intellectual disabilities (mentally retarded, socially deprived) snow ski, is to realize the capabilities of the human spirit. Disability (physical or mental) is no contraindication to participation in sport (Fig. 21).

Drug abuse
Drug abuse in sport, once widespread, is no longer tolerated, with severe penalties for guilty athletes. The International Olympic Committee has set the guidelines for other sport bodies. The banned drugs fall into the categories of stimulants narcotics, anabolic steroids, beta blockers (in general), diuretics, masking agents, peptide hormones, ethanol, tetrahydrocannabinol and phenobarbitol. Blood doping is illegal.

Drug effects   ***Anabolic steroids.*** These increase muscle mass and strength but adversely affect: the bone (enlarge) (Fig. 22); liver (failure or cancer); heart (cardiomegaly); testes (atrophy); skin (acne or hirsutism); kidney (failure); and personality ('roid rages').

Human growth hormone. This enhances lean body mass but causes acromegaly, cardiomyopathy and heart disease.

Amphetamines. These mask fatigue but may damage the CNS and heart.

Not only are drugs dangerous but they contravene the spirit of athletic competition.

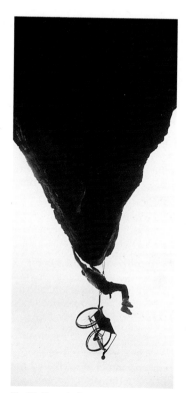

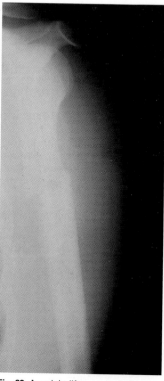

Fig. 21 Paraplegic rock climber (wheelchair attached).

Fig. 22 A weight lifter on anabolic steroids with a pathological fracture of the humerus.

5 / The female athlete

Today's female athlete is leaner, faster and stronger than ever, but there are some problems.

The female triad. Menstrual disorders, osteoporosis and eating disorders are together recognized as problems for the female athlete (Fig. 23).

Menstrual disorders

Delayed menarche

Incidence   The average age of menarche in non-athletes is 12–15 years and in athletes 13.5–15.5 years. For each year of training before menarche there is a delay of 5 months before the onset of menses in ballet dancers, gymnasts and long distance runners.

Treatment   This involves reducing the intensity and duration of training, increasing weight and encouraging balanced nutritional diets.

Exercise-associated amenorrhoea (EAA) (Fig. 24)

Incidence   Competitive training affects the menstrual cycle. In the general population 2–5% of women have amenorrhoea; in athletes the range is 3.4–66%. Oligomenorrhoea is seen in >30% of athletes.

Adverse effects   Normal levels of oestrogen are needed to maintain bone density in trabecular and cortical bone.

Short-term effects. Consequences of decreased bone mineral density (BMD) are in the short term an increase in stress fractures.

Long-term effects. Osteoporotic fractures occur before menopause.

Treatment   History, physical examination, full blood count, urinalysis, thyroid screen and hormone levels, altered training schedule and oestrogen therapy.

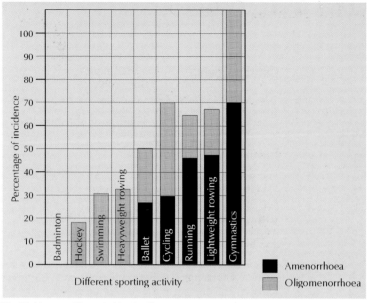

Fig. 23 Menstrual irregularities in elite sportswomen.

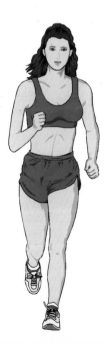

Altered body fat (<22% body weight)
•
Intensity of training
•
Intensive training before menarche
•
Younger age of athletes
•
Increased endorphin levels and other hormonal changes
•
Psychological and physiological stresses
•
Nulliparity
•
Menstrual irregularities prior to training
•
Diets low in protein, fat and calories

Fig. 24 Predisposing factors for EAA.

Osteoporosis

Definition   Osteoporosis is a decrease in bone mass and strength which leads to an increased incidence of fractures, especially of the vertebral body, neck of femur, humerus and wrist (Fig. 25).

Cause   It is a result of:

- hypo-oestrogenic state seen in EAA which has reduced BMD
- reduced dietary calcium.

Prevention   **Primary prevention:** includes increased dietary calcium (to 1500 mg/day) and reducing the amount of exercise.

Secondary prevention: is with oestrogen therapy and/or the combined oral contraceptive pill, then hormone replacement therapy at the time of menopause (or within 5–6 years) as well as calcium supplements.

Stress fractures

Definition   These are fractures caused by repetitive submaximal loads (fatigue type) or normal stress on deficient bone (insufficiency type).

Risk factors   Amenorrhoea/oligomenorrhoea/reduced dietary calcium/lower oral contraceptive use.

Sites
- Tibia, fibula in runners.
- Inferior pubic ramus in marathon runners.
- Pars interarticularies L5 vertebra in gymnasts and cricketers.

Clinical features   There is a history of repeated activity with pain before, during and after exercise. The area is swollen, warm and tender.

Treatment   This involves an elastic bandage or splintage, rest and avoidance/modification of training until healed.

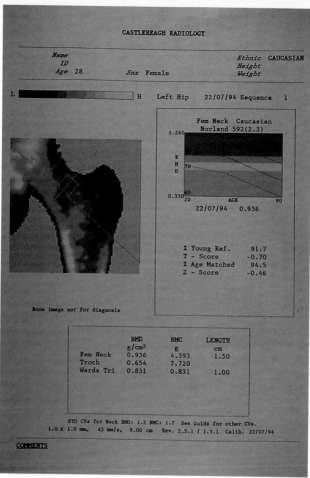

Fig. 25 A dual energy X-ray absorption (DEXA) bone mineral density scan can detect subtle decreases in bone mass.

Eating disorders

Prevalence The prevalence in the normal population is 0.5–1% of women. In competitive athletes it is 6.5%.

Athletes at risk Athletes most at risk are gymnasts, ballet dancers and skaters.

Leanness forms a subjective part of the scoring with an extreme desire to be thin and with a distorted body image (individuals perceive themselves as being overweight).

Types of disorder Disorders include:

- *Anorexia nervosa* (self-starvation with severe weight loss)
- *Bulimia nervosa* (as above but weight normal, self-purging and binge eating)
- *Eating disorder not otherwise specified* (average weight, may binge eat but do not purge).

Clinical features There are certain well-described warning symptoms and signs (Fig. 26). Treatment is difficult and not very successful. Intensive psychotherapy is necessary and hospitalization (where 35% loss of body weight has occurred). Mortality is 6%. Complications include nutritional deficiencies, decreased immune function, electrolyte distubances, psychiatric problems, amenorrhoea and decreased bone density.

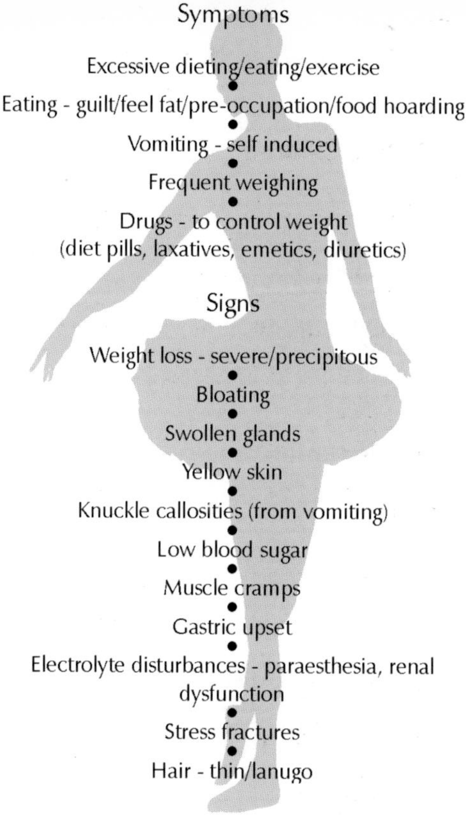

Symptoms

Excessive dieting/eating/exercise

Eating - guilt/feel fat/pre-occupation/food hoarding

Vomiting - self induced

Frequent weighing

Drugs - to control weight
(diet pills, laxatives, emetics, diuretics)

Signs

Weight loss - severe/precipitous

Bloating

Swollen glands

Yellow skin

Knuckle callosities (from vomiting)

Low blood sugar

Muscle cramps

Gastric upset

Electrolyte disturbances - paraesthesia, renal
dysfunction

Stress fractures

Hair - thin/lanugo

Fig. 26 Eating disorders signpost.

Iron deficiency

Strenuous exercise lowers plasma iron levels as there is increased red blood cell breakdown. This is called sports anaemia. The athlete can be iron deficient with or without anaemia.

Contraception

No sport precludes the use of any particular contraceptive measure.

Menstruation and performance

It appears that conditioning minimizes the adverse effects of menstruation on performance. Long-duration events (rowing, cycling) are affected by hormonal cycling (Fig. 27).

Vaginitis

This should be diagnosed and treated vigorously to minimize interference with performance.

Pregnancy

Exercise in pregnancy may be beneficial in normal-risk pregnancies.

Musculoskeletal injuries

The female athlete is prone to certain injuries. These are:

- paronychia
- rotator cuff tendinitis (Fig. 28)
- patellofemoral tracking problems
- anterior cruciate ligament tears, ankle impingement (including in plantar flexion, os trigonum) and forefoot problems (bunions and hammer toes)
- spondylolysis and vertebral body apophysitis (Fig. 29) in gymnasts and skaters.

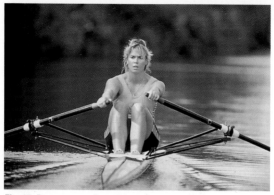

Fig. 27 Rowers are affected by hormonal cycling.

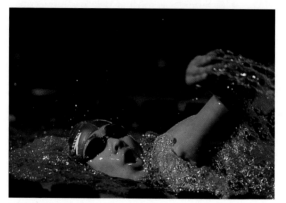

Fig. 28 Freestyle stroke can cause rotator cuff tendinitis.

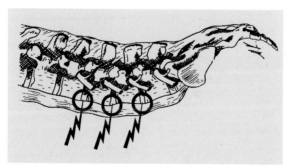

Fig. 29 Vertebral ring apophysis injury at the area of attachment of the anterior longitudinal ligament.

6 / Injuries of the shoulder

The shoulder is the most mobile of joints and yet is structurally insecure.

Instability

Classification

Instability occurs with the shoulder completely out of its socket (*dislocation*), or with lesser degrees of slipping where the shoulder is not completely out of joint (*subluxation*). Instability is usually anterior or antero-inferior (seldom posterior or multidirectional).

Anterior instability

Mechanism of injury

The shoulder is most at risk for anterior instability when the arm is placed in abduction/external rotation (such as a fall on the outstretched hand or tackling a player). In other cases there is no traumatic event but involvement in upper limb overhead sports.

Clinical features

Frank anterior dislocation is obvious (Fig. 30) but instability can have slipping; pain with the arm in abduction/external rotation; apprehension using the arm overhead or a 'dead arm' feeling with a tackle or overhead action.

Treatment

Acute dislocation. Exclude nerve or vascular injury. Closed reduction (Figs 31 & 32) can be achieved in the emergency room. In cases (where there is a high risk of recurrence) an acute arthroscopic assessment and repair may be offered. The risk of recurrent instability is highest (60–85%) in patients younger than 25 years returning to violent contact or upper limb sports.

Recurrent dislocation. For those patients with recurrent instability, treatment is to modify or avoid the known precipitating event; undergo physiotherapy rehabilitation programme or consider a reconstruction of the shoulder.

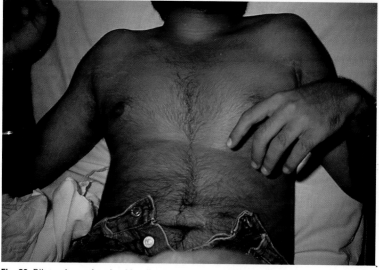

Fig. 30 Bilateral anterior shoulder dislocations with typical posture.

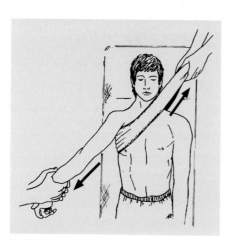

Fig. 31 Classical method of reducing anterior shoulder dislocation.

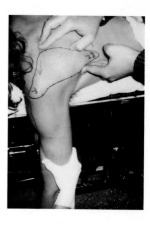

Fig. 32 New scapular rotation technique is less traumatic (Photograph courtesy of Dr J. French).

Posterior instability

Mechanism of injury
Traumatic posterior dislocations are uncommon (4%) and occur in electrocution or grand mal convulsion. Posterior subluxation is being recognized more frequently, occurring in athletes involved in sports such as baseball.

Clinical features
The diagnosis is often missed. The patients may have pain and an inability to externally rotate the arm (Fig. 33). The axillary X-ray view is diagnostic (Fig. 34).

Treatment
Reduce early. If the dislocation is longer-standing or a large portion of the humeral head is damaged, then surgical reconstruction of the humeral head is required; rarely total shoulder replacement.

Multidirectional instability

Clinical features
Signs of ligamentous laxity are present (Fig. 35). Patients often have pain and weakness with a shoulder that subluxes anteriorly, posteriorly (Fig. 36) and inferiorly. Examination shows a loose shoulder with a sulcus sign on inferior stress testing (Fig. 37, p. 36).

Treatment
The majority of patients will respond to physiotherapy. Rarely surgery is indicated.

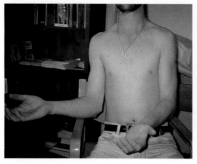

Fig. 33 Posterior shoulder dislocation: arm is locked in internal rotation.

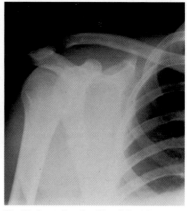

Fig. 34 Posterior shoulder dislocation (symmetrical ice-cream cone appearance of humeral head).

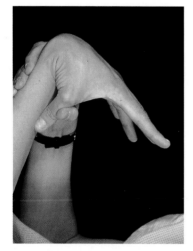

Fig. 35 Classical sign of ligamentous laxity.

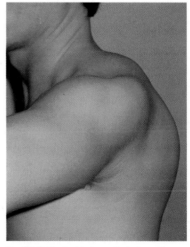

Fig. 36 Patient able to posteriorly sublux his shoulder.

Tendinitis and impingement

Mechanism of injury

Tendinitis can occur due to rotator cuff overload/fatigue, trauma, and age-related degenerative changes. Crowding of the cuff tendons in the subacromial space leads to impingement.

Clinical features

There is pain that is aggravated by overhead activities. Night pain occurs in advanced cases. Tenderness is over the greater tuberosity and impingement signs are present (Fig. 38). X-rays may show an anterior acromial spur.

Treatment

An injection of corticosteroid and local anaesthetic into the subacromial space is often diagnostic, and therapeutic. Treatment involves activity modification, NSAIDs, and physiotherapy. Consider surgery in 6 months.

Rotator cuff tears

Mechanism of injury

These injuries (Fig. 39) occur: in the younger patient from trauma; in the older patient from underlying degenerative changes.

Clinical features

Pain occurs with overhead use of the arm and at night. There may be weakness; only massive rotator cuff tears cause loss of active range of motion. X-rays often show an acromial spur. Investigations include either an arthrogram, ultrasound or magnetic resonance imaging (MRI).

Treatment

In the younger patient surgery is indicated. In the older patient a short trial of activity modification, NSAIDS, physiotherapy and corticosteroid injection is reasonable, and later surgery.

Acromioclavicular joint injuries

Mechanism of injury

These injuries are usually related to a fall on to the point of the shoulder. Pain, tenderness and deformity ensue.

Treatment

RICE (rest, ice, compression, elevation) and a sling, with surgery for major dislocations in active patients (Fig. 40).

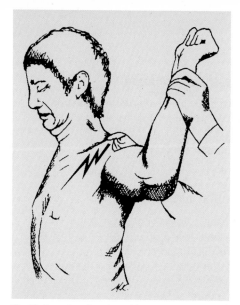

Fig. 37 Apprehension sign with anterior shoulder subluxation.

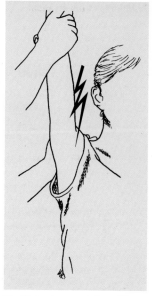

Fig. 38 Impingement sign with forward flexion.

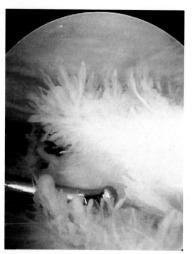

Fig. 39 Rotator cuff tear (at arthroscopy).

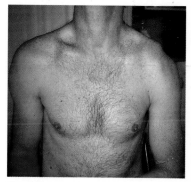

Fig. 40 Complete acromioclavicular dislocation.

Labral tears and loose bodies

Mechanism of injury
These are often associated with direct trauma or instability.

Clinical features
There is pain, clicking or locking. Instability may be present. Diagnosis is difficult (Fig. 41).

Treatment
Arthroscopy.

Outer clavicular osteolysis

Mechanism of injury
Injury results from a direct blow or fall but is often found in individuals who work out in the gymnasium on overhead machines or benchpresses.

Clinical features
X-ray examination shows irregularity of the outer clavicle with osteolysis.

Sternoclavicular dislocation

Mechanism of injury
Usually, dislocation is caused by a fall on to the side with another player falling on top causing compression of the shoulder. Dislocation can be anterior or posterior.

Clinical features
Anterior dislocation has a painful prominence (Fig. 42); posterior dislocation may cause pressure on structures in the neck with dysphagia, dyspnoea or great vessel compression (this can be a surgical emergency). X-rays are often difficult to interpret. A CT scan may be necessary.

Treatment
Anterior dislocations may be reduced closed or left. Posterior dislocations should be reduced urgently if there is compromise of mediastinal structures.

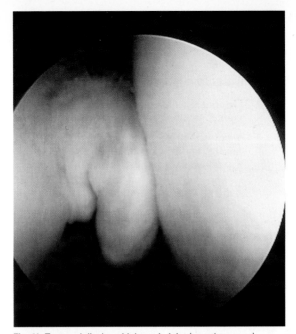

Fig. 41 Torn and displaced labrum in joint (at arthroscopy).

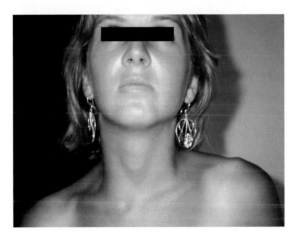

Fig. 42 Anterior sternoclavicular dislocation.

Muscle ruptures

Rupture usually occurs on contraction of muscle against an unexpected resistance. Muscles include:

- pectoralis major
- long head of biceps (Fig. 43)
- subscapularis.

Biceps tendinitis

Inflammation of the biceps tendon may occur with anterior instability or rotator cuff tears.

Nerve injuries

Mechanism of injury

Injuries to nerves can be secondary to instability or result from direct trauma. Traction to the arm can causes a neuropraxia. Nerves involved often include:

- circumflex axillary
- suprascapular
- musculocutaneous
- long thoracic (Fig. 44)
- radial.

Brachial plexus palsy (partial or complete) occurs with high-energy trauma.

Treatment

In most cases the injury is a neuropraxia and will recover with time. Electromyography (EMG) is recommended. Rarely, exploration and repair are required.

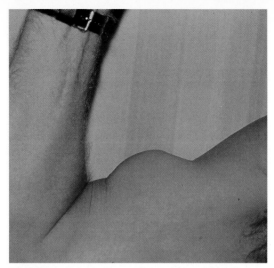

Fig. 43 'Pop-eye' appearance of ruptured long head of biceps.

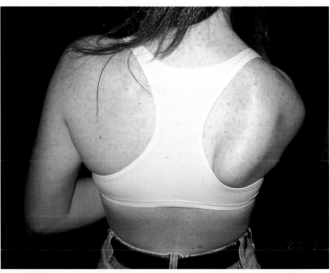

Fig. 44 Winging of scapula (serratus anterior weakness from long thoracic nerve palsy).

7/ Injuries of the elbow

Most elbow injuries are the result of overuse activities involved in upper limb sports.

Osteochondritis dissecans

Mechanism of injury
The aetiology is a combination of vascular and microtraumatic factors seen in throwing-type sports or gymnastics. There may have been a valgus or hyperextension load applied to the arm.

Clinical features
There is an insidious onset of vague elbow pain; in the adolescent, locking or catching may also occur; in the adult, arthritic symptoms. X-rays may show diffuse fragmentation of the distal humeral epiphysis (Panner's disease) or an osteochondral fragment (Fig. 45).

Treatment
In the young patient with diffuse epiphyseal fragmentation (Panner's disease), rest and activity modification. Loose bodies may require fixation or removal. Arthritis in later years is treated with activity modification, NSAIDs and surgery.

Little league elbow

Mechanism of injury
Medial epicondyle avulsion or any number of conditions causing medial-sided elbow pain from a valgus force and resistance load on the flexor muscles.

Clinical features
There is medial-sided elbow pain on loading the flexor muscles (Fig. 46). X-rays may show a separation of the medial epiphysis from the distal humerus (Fig. 47).

Treatment
Rest and activity modification and rarely surgery.

Tennis elbow

Mechanism of injury
A lateral epicondylitis from repetitive use of the arm especially with a clenched fist. Most cases are not due to tennis.

Clinical features
There is local tenderness and pain with resisted and passive extension of the wrists.

Treatment
Rest, activity modification, NSAIDs and physiotherapy will relieve most cases. Changing the grip size of the tennis racquet should be considered (Fig. 48). Only in refractory cases is surgery indicated.

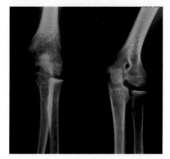

Fig. 45 Osteochondritis dissecans of distal humeral epiphysis (Panner's disease).

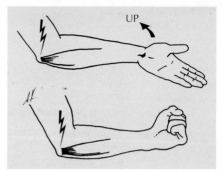

Fig. 46 Flexion load on forearm (with valgus force) causes medial elbow pain.

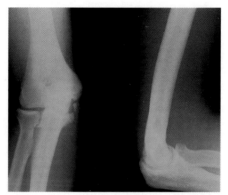

Fig. 47 Separation of medial humeral epiphysis.

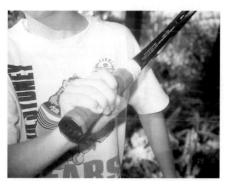

Fig. 48 Wrong grip size (here too big) may cause tennis elbow.

Golfer's elbow

Mechanism of injury

Patients are involved with racquet or club swinging and may jar the elbow or simply overuse the arm.

Clinical features

There is medial elbow pain with local tenderness and pain on loading the flexor muscles.

Treatment

Rest, activity modification, NSAIDs and physiotherapy; only rarely surgery.

Valgus extension overload: ulnar collateral ligament injuries

Mechanism of injury

Valgus stress on the elbow occurs with a throw. There may be a single throw or the condition may occur after repetitive throwing or occasionally a fall.

Clinical features

In the acute case there is local swelling and pain over the medial side or transient paraesthesia of the ulnar nerve. Valgus stress testing with the arm at 30° of flexion shows increased laxity and pain (Fig. 49). X-rays may show loose osseous bodies (Fig. 50).

Treatment

Rest, activity modification, NSAIDs and physiotherapy or later surgery.

Fractures/dislocation

Mechanism of injury

Usually a fall on to the outstretched hand or direct trauma.

Clinical features

With elbow dislocation there may be associated neurological (usually a neuropraxia) and/or vascular injury (Fig. 52). X-rays may show an obvious fracture or dislocation (Fig. 51). However, with fractures that are small or difficult to see the only clue may be the 'fat pad sign'.

Treatment

Reduction is a surgical emergency. Extra-articular fractures need reduction; intra-articular fractures need precise anatomic reduction.

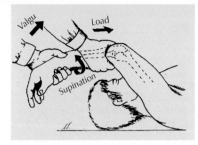

Fig. 49 Valgus stress testing of elbow will reproduce the pain.

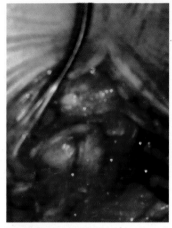

Fig. 50 Fracture radial head (at time of surgical fracture).

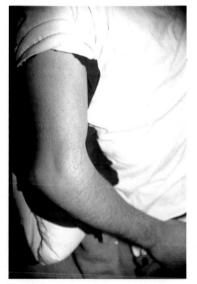

Fig. 51 Posterolateral elbow dislocation.

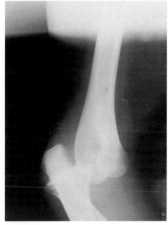

Fig. 52 Posterolateral elbow dislocation.

Loose bodies

Mechanism of injury
Most often, loose bodies (Fig. 53) arise as a consequence of old trauma, degenerative arthritis (Fig. 54) or osteochondritis dissecans.

Clinical features
Pain and locking are the predominant features.

Treatment
The symptoms of locking are treated by removal of the loose bodies. Treatment of the underlying condition is also required.

Ulnar nerve injuries

Mechanism of injury
Ulnar nerve injury most often occurs in throwing athletes from the excessive valgus load on the elbow during the cocking phase of throwing and is rarely due to direct trauma. Previous trauma with resultant cubitus valgus predisposes the elbow to ulnar nerve problems.

Clinical features
Tingling and numbness in the distribution of the ulnar nerve (Fig. 55). This may occur during or after throwing a ball or with prolonged elbow flexion.

Treatment
Correction of throwing style associated with forearm strengthening is recommended. If the problem persists or there is weakness and wasting, then surgery is indicated.

Osteoarthritis

Mechanism of injury
Causes include trauma (both major and repetitive micro), osteochondritis dissecans and associated synovial disease such as chondrometaplasia.

Clinical features
Pain, stiffness and locking. X-rays demonstrate osteophytes and loss of joint space (Fig. 56, p. 48).

Treatment
Rest, physiotherapy, NSAIDs with modification of activity and later surgery.

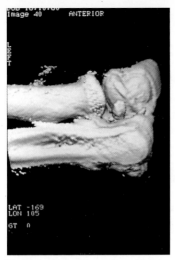

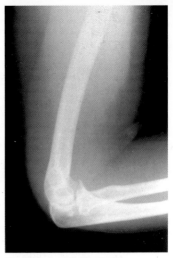

Fig. 53 Loose bodies on ulnar side joint (CT reconstruction).

Fig. 54 Osteoarthritis of elbow as source of loose bodies.

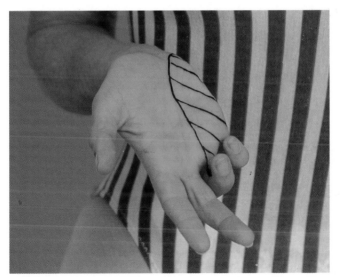

Fig. 55 Ulnar nerve hand signs (numbness and clawing).

Distal biceps rupture

Mechanism of injury
Rupture occurs with a sudden extension force while contracting the biceps. Pain and weakness result.

Clinical features
There is sudden onset of pain with swelling in the forearm. Weakness of flexion is evident. X-rays are often normal.

Treatment
In most cases surgical repair is indicated.

Distal triceps rupture

This results from sudden forced extension while the elbow is being flexed (Fig. 57). In most cases surgical repair is indicated.

Nerve compression syndromes (cubital tunnel, pronator syndrome, posterior interosseous, anterior interosseous)

Mechanism of injury
Occasionally there is a fracture around the elbow. In many cases no major trauma has occurred and the condition is of gradual onset. (There may be localized ganglia or enlarged bursae about the joint.)

Clinical features
There are localized sensory or motor changes. Careful clinical examination is needed to detect partial changes (e.g. with anterior interosseous nerve injury there is loss of deep flexors and small muscles of the hand without loss of flexor superficialis and wrist flexors). The 'OK' sign (Fig. 58) demonstrates functional flexor pollicis longus (FPL) and flexor digitorum profundus (FDP) muscles. If the 'OK' sign is lost, X-ray and nerve conduction studies are indicated.

Treatment
Early diagnosis is important. Many nerve injuries are neuropraxias and will resolve. If the nerve conduction study shows compression, then exploration is indicated.

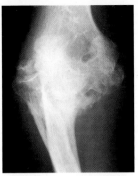

Fig. 56 Advanced osteoarthritis of elbow (ankylosis).

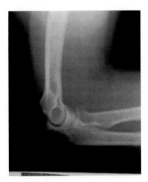

Fig. 57 Distal triceps avulsion (lower humerus).

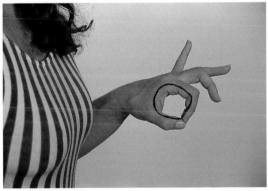

Fig. 58 'OK' sign intact (no nerve palsy).

8 / Injuries of the hand and wrist

Injuries of the hand and wrist are common in sport but often ignored during competition, with long-term consequences.

Carpal tunnel syndrome

Mechanism of injury

This is a common injury in tennis players and cyclists. The median nerve is compressed within the carpal tunnel (Fig. 59), producing pain and paraesthesia (radial $3\frac{1}{2}$ digits), often at night, and clumsiness.

Clinical features

There is decreased median nerve sensation, irritability of the nerve (positive Tinel's and Phalen's test) and later muscle weakness/wasting (test abductor pollicis brevis). Nerve conduction tests should be carried out if the diagnosis is in doubt.

Treatment

Includes splinting, NSAID gel, precise steroid injection but often surgical release (may be arthroscopic) before muscle wasting occurs.

Guyon's canal syndrome (handlebar palsy)

This syndrome is seen in cyclists (often coexisting with carpal tunnel syndrome) where the ulnar nerve is compressed in its canal over the wrist (Fig. 60). Treatment is similar to that of carpal tunnel syndrome but surgery is less frequently required.

Tendinitis

De Quervain's tendinitis. Injury results from compression of the extensor pollicis brevis (EPB) and abductor pollicis longus (APL) tendons in the first extensor compartment of the wrist (Fig. 61). The condition is seen in racket sports and golf. Treatment is rest, splint or surgical release.

Intersection syndrome ('squeakers'). The syndrome is seen in oarsmen where the tendons APL/EPB intersect extensor carpi radialis longis (ECRL)/extensor carpi radialis brevis (ECRB) and cause inflammation (Fig. 61). Treatment is rest, splint, NSAIDs and rarely surgery.

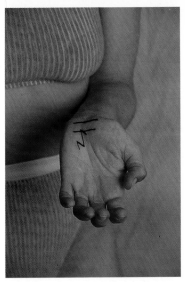

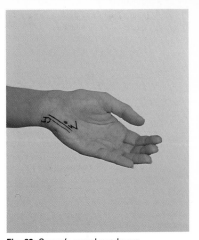

Fig. 60 Guyon's canal syndrome—compression of ulnar nerve at wrist.

Fig. 59 Carpal tunnel syndrome—nerve compressed by transverse carpal ligament.

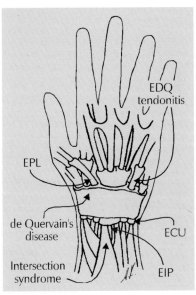

Fig. 61 Common sites of tendinitis over back of hand and wrist.

Fractures

Distal radius fracture

Fracture of the distal end of the radius results from a fall on to the outstretched hand or a directed blow. There are pain, tenderness and deformity (dinner-fork usually). The X-ray picture is typical.

A poorer prognosis occurs with comminuted fractures into the joint (Fig. 62).

Treatment Closed reduction is best, but displaced intra-articular fractures may require surgical fixation.

Scaphoid fracture

This is the most common carpal fracture (seen in contact sports such as football) and is often wrongly diagnosed as a 'sprained wrist'. There is snuff box tenderness or pain with axial compression along the thumb (scaphoid impaction test (SIT); Fig. 63).

Treatment Treatment is difficult. A non-displaced fracture requires a thumb spica (6 weeks or until union); a displaced fracture (Fig. 64) will require surgical fixation. The precarious blood supply (enters distally) predisposes to non-union and avascular necrosis (long-term OA). Elite athletes may prefer early surgical fixation.

Other fractures

Hook of hamate fracture. This injury typically occurs when a golf swing makes violent contact with the ground (or from repeated trauma in baseball) with point tenderness. The X-ray appearance (carpal tunnel view) is shown in Figure 65.

Bennett's fracture. This is an intra-articular fracture of the base of the 1st metacarpal. Closed reduction with percutaneous K-wire fixation is required.

Fractures of the phalanges and metacarpals.
These fractures are not uncommon and in general can be treated by closed reduction and splintage (otherwise percutaneous K-wire fixation).

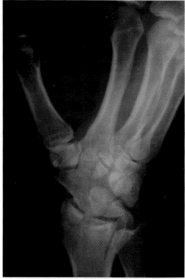

Fig. 62 Intra-articular fracture of the distal radius carries poor prognosis.

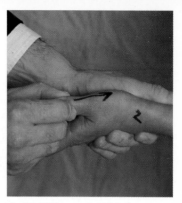

Fig. 63 SIT for scaphoid injury.

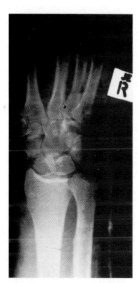

Fig. 64 Displaced fracture of waist of scaphoid.

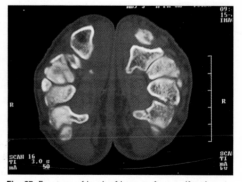

Fig. 65 Fracture of hook of hamate from golf swing.

Mallet (baseball) finger

Mechanism of injury
A blow to the tip of the finger forces the distal phalanx into flexion, avulsing the extensor insertion (Fig. 66). This commonly occurs whilst catching the ball in cricket, baseball and basketball.

Clinical features
There is a flexion deformity of the distal interphalangeal (DIP) joint with pain and swelling. X-rays may show a bone fragment.

Treatment
Closed rupture (without bone fragment) requires splintage of the DIP joint in full extension for a minimum of 6 weeks (continuously). Surgical repair is indicated when there is a displaced bone fragment or subluxed joint.

Flexor digitorum profundus tendon avulsion (jersey finger)

Mechanism of injury
Injury, usually to the ring finger, results from active flexion against distal interphalangeal extension (whilst holding on to another player's rugger jersey).

Clinical features
There is loss of active flexion of the DIP joints (stabilize proximal interphalangeal joint (PIP) and request flexion of DIP), tenderness and swelling along finger flexor sheath or palm (feel stump). X-rays may show a bone fragment (Fig. 67).

Treatment
Primary surgical repair is difficult and best not delayed. Two-stage reconstruction is needed in delayed cases.

Boutonnière deformity

Mechanism of injury
There is a closed rupture of the central slip of the extensor (or middle phalanx) or open injury.

Clinical features
There is PIP flexion and DIP hyperextension with tenderness and swelling over the central slip and an inability to strongly extend the PIP joint (Fig. 68).

Treatment
Splint closed ruptures (at least 6 weeks). Surgery is required for an open injury. Later deformities are difficult to treat; surgery is often not useful.

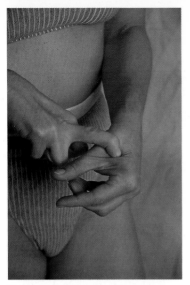

Fig. 66 Mallet deformity of long finger.

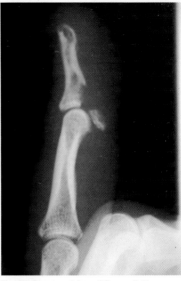

Fig. 67 Bony avulsion of flexor digitorum profundus tendon.

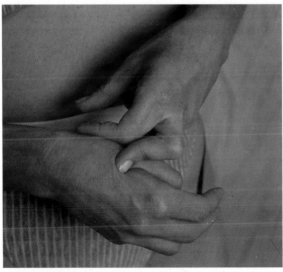

Fig. 68 Boutonnière deformity of long finger.

Proximal interphalangeal joint injuries

PIP joint injury (Fig. 69) often results in stiffness. Collateral ligament injuries occur from a jammed finger (buddy strap for 3–6 weeks). Radial collaterals may require surgical repair. Dislocations are common (especially dorsal—reduce and buddy strap; rotatory type may be irreducible and require open reduction). Fractures with dislocations are difficult to reduce and often require open reduction/fixation (volar plate interposition).

Metacarpophalangeal (MCP) dislocations

These are usually easily reduced by closed technique. If dorsal, the metacarpal head may buttonhole into the palm (locked by the volar plate). On X-ray examination, sesamoids will lie over the joint and the skin is puckered. Open reduction is then required.

Skier's thumb (gamekeeper's thumb)

Mechanism of injury

Injury results from sudden forced radial deviation of the thumb proximal phalanx on the metacarpal, commonly from skiing and football.

Clinical features

There is ulnar-sided pain, swelling and joint instability (Fig. 70). X-ray examination often shows an avulsed fragment from the base of the proximal phalanx.

Treatment

Splint partial tears (Fig. 71); surgically repair complete tears.

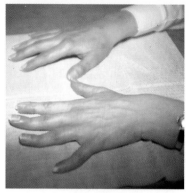

Fig. 69 Multiple finger (PIP) dislocations—careful attention required.

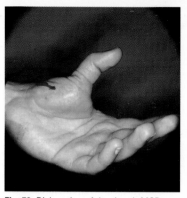

Fig. 70 Dislocation of the thumb MCP joint.

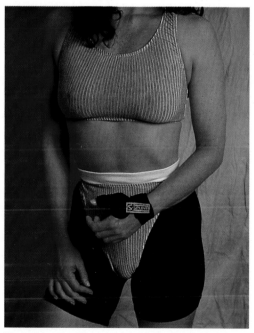

Fig. 71 Most partial tears can be treated with a splint.

Triangular fibrocartilage complex (TFCC) tears

Mechanism of injury
Injury is cased by a fall on to the outstreched hand or resisted rotation of the hand on the forearm. This is a common cause of ulnar-sided wrist pain that is exacerbated by gripping.

Clinical features
Rotation of the forearm causes clicking and pain. There is tenderness over the ulnar head and styloid.

Treatment
If the condition is still symptomatic after rest and splintage, consider arthroscopic debridement of the tear (Fig. 72), repair or reconstruction of the TFCC.

Scapholunate (and lunotriquetral) ligament tears

Mechanism of injury
Such tears result from a fall on to the outstretched wrist. Diagnosis is often delayed.

Clinical features
- In scapholunate tears pain and clunking occur with pressure over the scaphoid tubercle when the wrist is taken from ulnar to radial deviation (Watson's test).
- In lunotriquetral tears there is a positive ballotment test (Fig. 73).

Advanced osteoarthritis may occur. X-rays may demonstrate an increasing gap between the carpal bones (Terry Thomas sign) or joint incongruity indicating complete rupture and carpal subluxation (dorsal/volar intercalated segmental instability). Gross injury results in dislocation (Fig. 74).

Treatment
Repair of completely ruptured ligaments in a new injury, or later reconstruction.

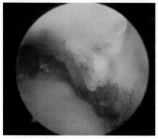

Fig. 72 Arthroscopic debridement of TFCC tear.

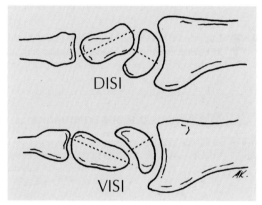

Fig. 73 Carpal ligament tears (DISI—scapholunate; VISI—lunotriquetral) with subluxation.

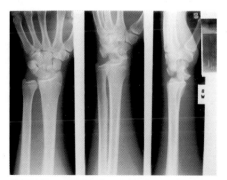

Fig. 74 Trans-scapho (scaphoid fracture) perilunate dislocation of wrist.

9 / Injuries of the hip, thigh and pelvis

Injuries of this region can be serious.

Contusion of quadriceps (corked thigh, charley horse)

Mechanism of injury
This is the result of a direct blow during contact sports. It occurs at the musculotendinous junction of rectus femoris.

Clinical features
There is pain, stiffness, a limp, progressive swelling and bruising.

Treatment
Includes RICE (rest, ice, compression, elevation). Early attention is required because of the risk of myositis ossificans. Beware of the risk of a compartment syndrome.

Keep the knee flexed and well padded.

Myositis ossificans traumatica

Mechanism of injury
A severe contusion or tear that occurs to the quadriceps may lead to haematoma formation followed by acute inflammation. Fibroblasts may form osteoid (Fig. 75).

Treatment
RICE and strict rest. Occasionally drainage of the haematoma is required, or excision after 12 months.

Quadriceps strains and rupture

Mechanism of injury
This is a result of severe contraction when either accelerating or kicking.

Clinical features
There is localized tenderness or a defect (Fig. 76). The pain is exacerbated by resistance of hip flexion in extension and full knee flexion in a prone position.

Avulsion of the iliac spines (anterior-superior and inferior)

This injury is caused by sudden severe contracture of rectus femoris (in soccer players) or sartorius muscle (Fig. 77). Players tend to be in their mid-teens. The X-ray appearance is typical.

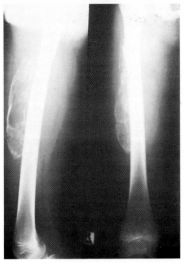

Fig. 75 Myositis ossificans of quadriceps.

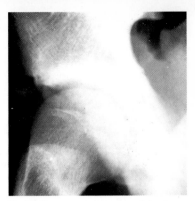

Fig. 77 Bony rectus femoris avulsion from anterior inferior iliac spine.

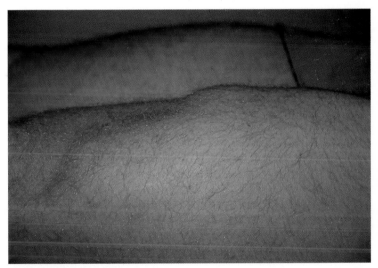

Fig. 76 Defect from quadriceps rupture.

Ischial apophysitis (weaver's bottom, ischial bursitis) and avulsion

Mechanism of injury This is a result of excessive running, especially in adolescents. Repetitive strain is put upon the apophysis, compounded by tight hamstrings. Severe contracture of the hamstrings (in the skeletally immature) may avulse the tuberosity (Figs 78 & 79).

Groin strain (adductor strain)

Mechanism of injury This occurs in sports where cutting, side-stepping, or pivoting are required (seen in soccer players). There is violent external rotation, with the leg in a widely abducted position. Well-localized tenderness is a feature.

Hip pointer

A direct blow to the iliac crest in contact sports, also known as iliac crest contusion, may result in painful periostitis or exostosis formation. Exclude avulsion of the anterior inferior iliac spine in adolescents by X-ray examination. Treat with RICE, NSAIDs, stretching, padding and sometimes a steroid injection.

Trochanteric bursitis

Mechanism of injury This is the result of increased shear stress created by the iliotibial tract over the trochanter (Figs 80 & 81). It is often associated with a broad pelvis, a large quadriceps angle and leg length discrepancies.

Clinical features There is pain over the lateral aspect of the thigh when lying on the affected side. Abducting against resistance in the internally rotated and adducted position exacerbates the pain.

Treatment Includes RICE, physical therapy with stretching of the iliotibial band, and correction of any leg length discrepancy and/or abnormal running style. Steroid injections can be useful, but surgery is rarely required.

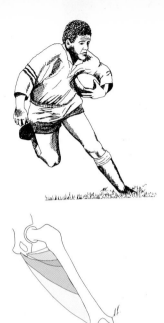

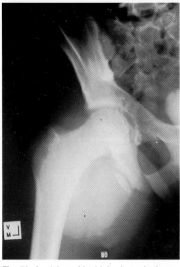

Fig. 79 Avulsion of ischial tuberosity in an athlete after 1 year.

Fig. 78 Severe contracture will avulse the ischial tuberosity.

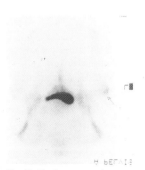

Fig. 80 Hot bone scan in trochanteric bursitis.

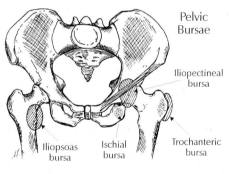

Pelvic Bursae

Iliopectineal bursa

Iliopsoas bursa

Ischial bursa

Trochanteric bursa

Fig. 81 Other sites of bursitis about the pelvis.

Hamstring strains

Mechanism of injury In the late swing phase of the gait cycle the hamstrings decelerate the limb. With sudden acceleration from stabilizing flexor to active extensor, strain is put on the hamstring muscles (Fig. 82).

Clinical features The short head of biceps femoris is commonly injured; a twinge or snap may be noted in this area. The patient experiences pain, swelling and may collapse in the sprinting motion.

Treatment Includes RICE and physical therapy. Recovery is slow; rehabilitation and an elastic stocking are used.

Snapping hip

Injury results from repetitive rubbing of the capsule in running or ballet. This can involve the iliopsoas tendon or the iliotibial band. There is anteromedial hip pain.

Hip joint strain (pericapsulitis, synovitis, irritable hip)

Mechanism of injury This may be due to a direct blow, twisting injury, or from overuse. There is inflammation of the lining or a strain of capsular ligaments (Fig. 83).

Clinical features There is a pain in the groin, which may radiate into the thigh. The most comfortable position is flexion, abduction and external rotation (Fig. 84).

Conjoint tendon strain of the hip

This results from stress on the abdominal musculature, especially when taking a mark in football or heading in soccer (Fig. 85).

Iliac crest apophysitis and avulsion

This is the result of repetitive stress in adolescence (seen with running, especially with a cross-over style of arm swing). Sudden contracture or direct blow may avulse or fracture the iliac crest.

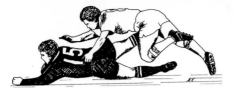

Fig. 82 Resisted hip extension will tear the hamstrings.

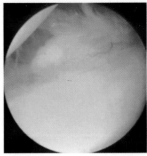

Fig. 83 Synovitis of the hip seen at arthroscopy.

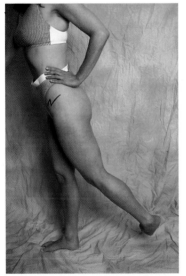

Fig. 84 Pain is reproduced in hip joint sprain by extension and internal rotation.

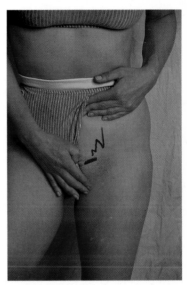

Fig. 85 Conjoint tendon strain of the hip.

Osteitis pubis/pubic symphysitis

This results from running, jumping and kicking, which place large shear stresses on the symphysis pubis. The condition is seen in hockey players, soccer players and runners.

It may lead to sub-periosteal damage and a subacute periostitis.

Obturator nerve entrapment

The mechanism of injury is unknown, but is probably related to scarring from previous injury.

Clinical features There is pain around the inner aspect of the thigh (Fig. 86).

Ilio-inguinal nerve entrapment

The mechanism of injury is unknown.

Clinical features There is pain and paraesthesia in the groin and hypo-aesthesia in the area about the inguinal ligament (Fig. 87). Occasionally there is tenderness at the exit point of the nerve from the muscle belly.

Labral tears

Mechanism of injury These are most commonly seen in dysplastic hips where there is abnormal shear and strain on the acetabular labrum and excessive twisting in sports.

Clinical features There is a sharp pain or catching sensation, superimposed on a dull ache. Tears are confirmed by arthrography or arthroscopy (usually in the posterior aspect of the hip joint) (Fig. 88).

Treatment Rest and surgical excision or repair.

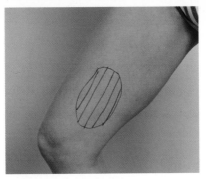

Fig. 86 Obturator nerve entrapment with sensory changes.

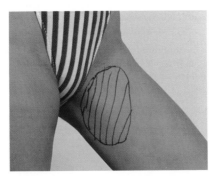

Fig. 87 Ilio-inguinal nerve entrapment with sensory changes.

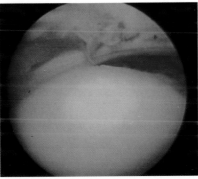

Fig. 88 Labral tear of hip (at arthroscopy).

Fractured hip: acute slip of the upper femoral epiphysis (SUFE)

Mechanism of injury
This occurs with a severe impact while the foot is planted and the hip twisted. It may occur in cross-country and downhill skiers from a low velocity fall ('skier's hip'). (Hip fracture may occur or SUFE in child.)

Clinical features
There is pain and an inability to bear weight, often associated with a shortening and external rotation in the hip. There may be a past history of ache or an antalgic gait with an acute or chronic slipped upper femoral epiphysis (Figs 89 & 90).

Treatment
Immediate immobilization is required, followed by urgent surgical stabilization and drainage of a capsular haematoma.

Stress fractures

Mechanism of injury
These are the result of repetitive impact in runners and occur most commonly in the proximal femur and femoral neck. X-rays show periosteal reaction and a bone scan is positive (Fig. 91).

Treatment
Rest, for a minimum of 2–3 months and then gradual return to activity.

Dislocation of the hip

Mechanism of injury
This is a result of a direct impact to the flexed knee and hip. It may be anterior or posterior.

Clinical features
There is pain and deformity with the leg in a flexed and internally rotated attitude (posterior dislocation) or externally rotated (anterior dislocation) (Fig. 92).

Treatment
Immobilization and urgent reduction of the hip (to reduce the likelihood of developing avascular necrosis).

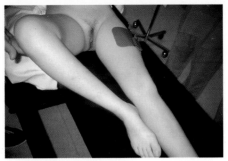

Fig. 89 SUFE—typically externally rotates with flexion of the hip.

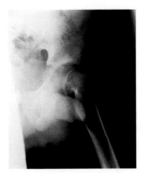

Fig. 90 SUFE.

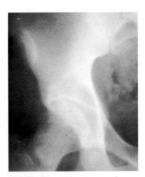

Fig. 91 Stress fractures of neck of femur.

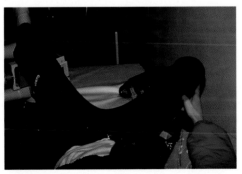

Fig. 92 Typical posture of right anterior hip dislocation.

Fractured femur and pelvis

Mechanism of injury
These injuries are a result of high-energy impact.

Clinical features
There is pain and deformity. It is important to assess for any neurological or vascular compromise. There are usually associated head, neck, chest and abdominal life-treatening injuries (Fig. 93).

Treatment
Resuscitate the patient with special attention to head injury status, immobilize the neck, exclude need for chest tube or peritoneal lavage/exploratory laparotomy. Maximize volume replacement (up to 40 units of blood can disappear into a fractured pelvis) and give adequate analgesia. Surgery is often necessary to stabilize the displaced fractures.

Avascular necrosis

Mechanism of injury
This results from a disrupted blood supply, from fracture, dislocation, or repetitive trauma.

Clinical features
There is pain, limitation of movement and an antalgic gait. X-rays reveal late changes. A bone scan and MRI are more sensitive in the early stages of this disorder.

Treatment
Rest with crutches, and management of the underlying disorder. Surgical decompression or a late reconstructive procedure may be required (Fig. 94).

Osteoarthritis of the hip

Athletes with extensive sport involvement have a 4- to 5-fold increase in OA of the hip (up to 8.5 if also an at-risk occupation) (Figs 95 & 96). Patients with hip replacements should not participate in impact sports.

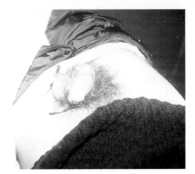

Fig. 93 Fractured pelvis. Note blood at tip of penis (ruptured urethra).

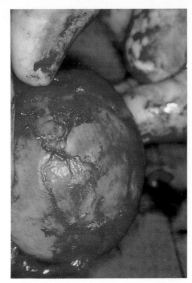

Fig. 94 Avascular necrosis of femoral head seen at surgery.

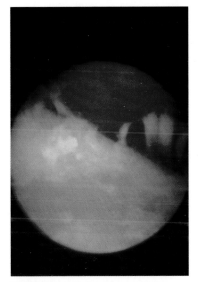

Fig. 95 Osteoarthritis of hip seen at arthroscopy.

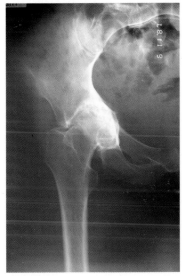

Fig. 96 Osteoarthritis of the hip.

10 / Injuries of the knee

The knee is the most commonly injured part of the body in sport.

Meniscal tears

Mechanism of injury

These usually occur when the flexed knee is externally rotated. The meniscus, usually the less mobile medial, is caught between the bone ends and torn (Fig. 97). Footballers and downhill snow skiers when changing direction are prone to this (Fig. 98).

Clinical features

There is joint line pain, instability, an effusion and locking of the knee. Apley's grinding test and McMurray's test may be positive. The tear often has a bucket handle or parrot beak configuration.

Treatment

This includes rest, ice, compression and elevation. Arthroscopic partial medial meniscectomy is indicated for a large tear which remains symptomatic. The meniscus is repaired when the tear is at the meniscocapular junction, especially in children (Fig. 99).

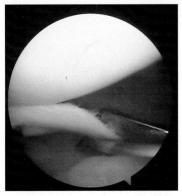

Fig. 97 Bucket-handle tear of the medial meniscus being resected.

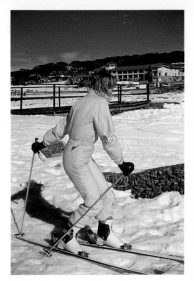

Fig. 98 A slow speed turn in snow skiing may cause a meniscal tear if the bindings do not release.

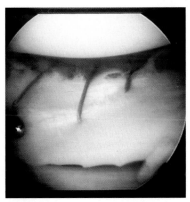

Fig. 99 Arthroscopic meniscal suture repair.

Tears of the anterior cruciate ligament

Mechanism of injury

The cruciate ligaments stabilize the knee. The anterior cruciate ligament (ACL) may rupture when a valgus/external rotating force is applied to the knee as when cutting in football or in the hyperflexed or hyperextended knee.

Clinical features

There is an immediate 'pop' sensation with a large effusion (blood) and pain (Fig. 100). The knee is unstable. Lachman's test (Fig. 101) is an accurate way of detecting an ACL tear (Fig. 102). The knee is flexed 30° and the upper tibia is found to move forward on the lower femur. The dynamic self-extension test and the pivot shift are also positive.

Treatment

Treatment includes intensive physiotherapy (hamstring strengthening) and later reconstruction of the ACL (using the middle third of the patellar tendon or part of the hamstrings) when the knee remains unstable in the young athlete.

The posterior cruciate ligament (PCL) is stronger and less commonly injured. Physiotherapy is required (avoid hamstring exercises) and seldom surgery. Osteoarthritis may secondarily develop.

Tears of the medial collateral ligament (MCL)

Mechanism of injury

MCL, partial or complete, tears are common. A valgus force produces the injury (Fig. 103).

Clinical features

There is medial knee pain and tenderness with opening of the flexed knee from an abduction load (almost painless with a complete tear). It may be associated with a medial meniscal tear and ACL rupture (O'Donoghue's unhappy triad).

Treatment

Partial and isolated complete tears need a brace and rehabilitation. Otherwise when in combination surgical repair is required.

Lateral collateral ligament tears (LCL) are less common and usually treated with a brace and rehabilitation.

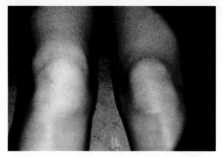

Fig. 100 A large immediate knee effusion will almost certainly be blood from an ACL rupture.

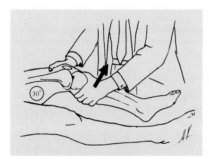

Fig. 101 Lachman's test.

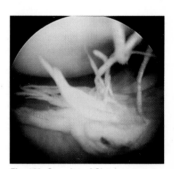

Fig. 102 Complete ACL tear at arthroscopy.

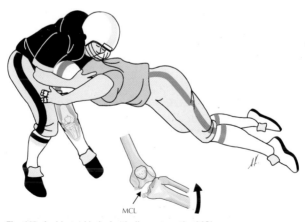

Fig. 103 A side tackle in football can tear the MCL.

MCL

Patellofemoral problems

The patellofemoral joint is prone to problems including maltracking (from malalignment causing subluxation or dislocation), chondromalacia patellae (CMP) and patellar tendonitis. These present as anterior knee pain.

Chondromalacia patellae

Clinical features There is softening of the patellar cartilage from direct contusion or malalignment (increased Q angle, see below) (Fig. 104). Young overweight girls with knock knees are susceptible. There is anterior knee pain with swelling and difficulty with prolonged sitting and using stairs.

Treatment Treatment includes symptomatic relief (RICE and analgesia) and quadriceps rehabilitation.

Maltracking of the patella

Clinical features Where there is an increased Q angle (angle between anterior superior iliac spine and tibial tubercle: normal $>15°$) and ligamentous laxity, subluxation may result (Fig. 105). There is anterior knee pain with instability. If the patella dislocates (Fig. 106), the patient falls to the ground.

Treatment Treatment includes activity modification, RICE, rebalancing of the extensor mechanism (stretching of tight lateral retinacular structures, strengthening of the vastus medialis: McConnell technique) and a patellar lift-off brace. Rarely, surgery is required to rebalance by releasing the tight lateral retinacular structures and reefing the lax medial.

Lateral patellar compression syndrome

In this syndrome, the Q angle is normal but lateral patellar retinacular structures are tight. Stretching or surgical release is required.

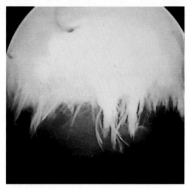

Fig. 104 Advanced (crabmeat) chondromalacia patellae at arthroscopy.

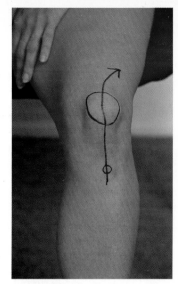

Fig. 105 Maltracking patellar (J-curve).

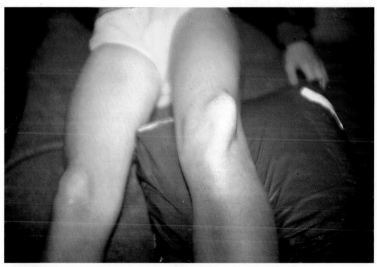

Fig. 106 A dislocated patella in a child (almost always laterally).

Iliotibial band friction syndrome

This occurs in runners (downhill) and cyclists from flicking of a tight iliotibial band across the lateral femoral condyle. Stretching or, rarely, excision of a posterior portion is required (Fig. 107).

Patellar tendinitis (jumper's knee, Sinding-Larsen–Johansson syndrome (SLJ))

Clinical features Jumping sports put a huge load on the extensor mechanism of the knee, usually at the lower pole of the patella, especially when there is excessive foot pronation. There is pain and crepitus in that area (Fig. 108).

Treatment Treatment includes activity modification, bracing (where there is ligamentous laxity), ultrasound and rarely surgical excision of the associated necrotic debris.

Osgood–Schlatter's disease. Here the lower end of the tendon is involved (see p. 111).

Patella alta/baja

The patella may be too high (alta) causing instability, or too low (baja) causing stiffness.

Plicas

Clinical features These are persistent vestigial folds of the synovium in the suprapatellar pouch, medial gutter or in front of the anterior cruciate ligament. They may become inflamed, thickened and fibrosed, causing pain and hamstring muscle spasm.

Treatment Rehabilitation is required and possibly arthroscopic surgical debridement (Fig. 109).

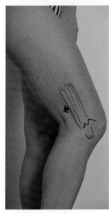

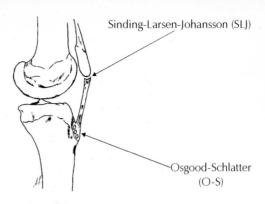

Sinding-Larsen-Johansson (SLJ)

Osgood-Schlatter
(O-S)

Fig. 108 A tendinitis of the upper patellar tendon is SLJ; of the lower, O–S (traction apophysitis).

Fig. 107 Iliotibial band friction syndrome with pain and tenderness over lateral knee.

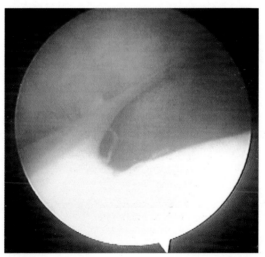

Fig. 109 A medial plica in a 16-year-old footballer which was symptomatic.

11 / Injuries of the foot, ankle and leg

Ankle sprains/instability

Mechanism of injury

Ankle sprains are the most common injury in sport and almost always involve the lateral ligament complex; usually the anterior talofibular ligament part (ATFL), and less frequently the calcaneofibular ligament (CFL), or in combination. Large athletes, those with high medial arches (pes cavus) and those who have had previous similar injury are at risk. High-top footwear and ankle splints may protect the ankle. Medial (deltoid) ligament injuries are rare. The ankle joint surface may also be damaged (transchondral fractures).

Clinical features

There is lateral ankle pain, swelling and a sense of instability. The anterior draw test is positive for ATFL injury (Fig. 110) and talar tilt (>45°) for CFL (Fig. 111). X-ray examinations are important to exclude fractures (e.g. Maisonneuve—high fibular fractures and syndesmotic rupture). Stress X-rays may be helpful.

Treatment

Acute injuries require RICE and protection (dorsiflexed in a splint to approximate the torn ATFL) (Fig. 112). Early rehabilitation (with peroneal strengthening and jogging in water) is essential. Surgical reconstruction of the ligaments is almost always reserved for chronic symptomatic instability (Fig. 113). Chondral damage may require arthroscopic attention.

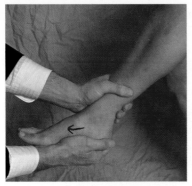

Fig. 110 Anterior draw test for ATFL tear.

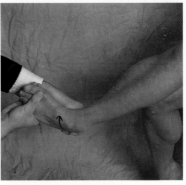

Fig. 111 Inversion test for CFL tear.

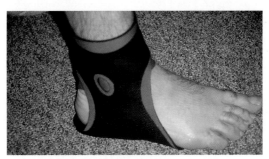

Fig. 112 Splint is used in rehabilitation.

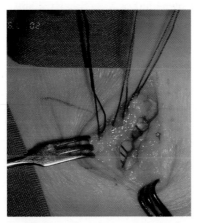

Fig. 113 Lateral ligament reconstruction for instability.

Fractures

Ankle

Mechanism of injury

Athletes may sprain or break their ankles. Fractures may involve the lateral, medial or posterior malleolus of the ankle joint. A fall with supination (or pronation) of the forefoot and eversion (or inversion) of the hindfoot can result in fracture. Well-fitted and firm ski boots have almost eliminated fractures from snow skiing.

Clinical features

There is pain, swelling and deformity. Skin problems (blisters and necrosis) may result from delayed reduction. A markedly displaced ankle fracture (Fig. 114) should be immediately reduced in casualty before theatre. X-ray examinations are essential. Carefully examine above (upper tibia, knee) and below (foot) to exclude associated fractures (Maisonneuve or Dupuytren's fracture) (Fig. 115).

Treatment

Early and accurate reduction with fixation are essential to avoid instability and secondary osteoarthritis.

Foot

Mechanism of injury

Fractures of the *calcaneus* result from a high fall and can be devastating. Problems include nerve (sural) and tendon (peroneal) entrapment, widened heel and subtalar OA.

Treatment

Accurate reduction (restoration of Böhler's angle) is important. Surgery is difficult. Early movement is important.

Talar fractures. Talar neck fractures may result in avascular necrosis of the talar body and need accurate reduction (Fig. 116).

Navicular fractures. These may be hairline/stress or comminuted. Non-union with pain may result.

Mid-foot (tarsometatarsal) fractures. These can be subtle and easily overlooked (Fig. 117). Reduction and fixation with K-wires is often required.

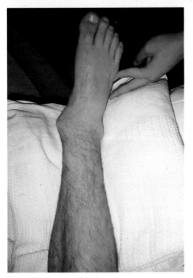

Fig. 114 Gross ankle fracture displacement.

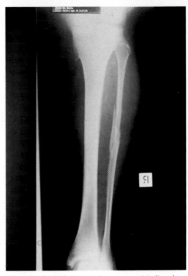

Fig. 115 (High) fibular fracture with (low) ankle diastasis injury (Maisonneuve fracture).

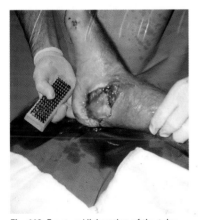

Fig. 116 Fracture/dislocation of the talus.

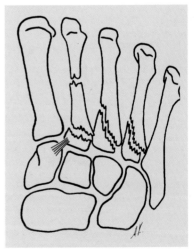

Fig. 117 Typical fracture patterns of the mid-foot (the second metatarsal is the keystone).

Achilles tendon rupture

Mechanism of injury
Violent contraction of the gastrocnemius-soleus muscle may rupture the Achilles tendon (TA). It occurs in the push-off phase of running or racket sports.

Clinical features
The patient often reports having been shot or kicked in the calf. There is pain and a gap in the tendon above the heel (prior to swelling). Simmond's test is diagnostic (Fig. 118).

Treatment
Surgical repair is best for the athlete (Fig. 119). Re-rupture may occur, therefore rehabilitation should be cautious.

Lesser degrees of injury of the Achilles tendon. These include:

- inflammation around the tendon (peritendinitis, seen in soccer)
- inflammation in the tendon (tendinitis; see painful arc sign, Fig. 120)
- partial rupture
- medial gastrocnemius strain (tennis leg).

Plantar fasciitis

Clinical features
This is a common cause of heel pain in athletes. There may be excessive pronation. Exclude stress fractures and Reiter's disease.

Treatment
Treatment is NSAIDs, a soft heel cup (orthotics) and stretching. Surgery is seldom useful.

Turf toe

Mechanism of injury
This is an American football injury. A forceful dorsiflexion of the 1st MTP joint produces a painful, swollen and stiff joint (Fig. 121).

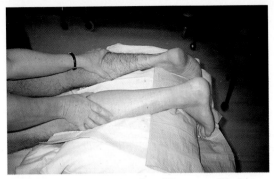

Fig. 118 Simmond's test: when the calf is squeezed the foot does not plantar flex (TA is ruptured).

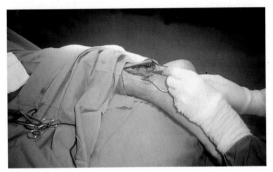

Fig. 119 Surgical repair is almost always required.

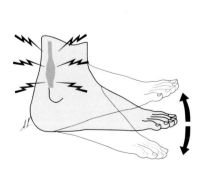

Fig. 120 Painful arc sign: pain site moves with foot (tendinitis); does not move (peritendinitis).

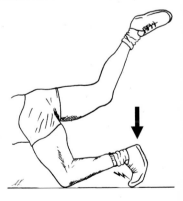

Fig. 121 Turf toe from forceful dorsiflexion of big toe.

Stress fractures

Mechanism of injury

These fractures result from repetitive submaximal loads applied to the foot, ankle or leg; the hallmark of intensive training schedules. They are not uncommon in soldiers, long distance runners and female athletes (in presence of menstrual disorders and osteoporosis).

Clinical features

Diagnosis can be difficult. Examine for pronated feet and marked external tibial torsion.

Common sites include the distal tibia (in runners), talus (dome), calcaneus (recruits), navicular (basketballers), metatarsals (neck in distance runners, base in ballet dancers) and phalanx (proximal big toe).

There is pain and localized tenderness, which, partially relieved by rest, is typical. X-rays do not always show the typical transverse fracture (beware the 'dreaded black line' of impending complete fracture). Bone scans are diagnostic (Fig. 122). MRI is useful.

Treatment

Most heal with rest, immobilization and cross-training. Avoid impact work and acquire better absorptive sports shoes (Fig. 123). After 6 months, surgery may be considered (with bone grafting). Female athletes may require hormone therapy.

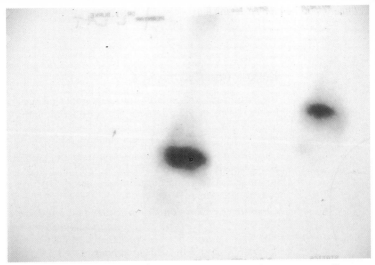

Fig. 122 Hot bone scan reveals stress fracture of *lower* tibia (X-ray was normal).

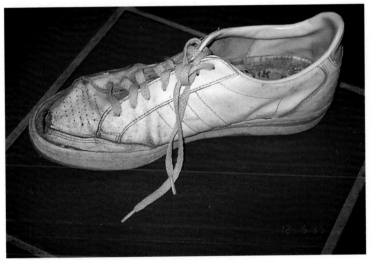

Fig. 123 Worn-out sports shoes: seen with stress fractures.

Compartment syndrome

Mechanism of injury Increased pressure within a muscle compartment can be disastrous, leading to necrosis, contracture and a useless limb.

The acute situation. This is well described (inordinate amount of pain, paraesthesia and pain on active/passive movement of that muscle) and *must not* be missed. Measuring intracompartmental pressures is courting disaster.

Chronic (or exertional) compartment syndrome. This may be subtle and result from prolonged running. The muscles have been over-worked and have swollen. The extensor and flexor compartments of the leg are aften involved.

Clinical features There is crescendo exertional pain relieved by rest. Stress fractures, periostitis (posteromedial tibia, shin splints) and popliteal artery entrapment (calf claudication) should be excluded.

Treatment Includes activity modification, NSAIDs, a medial heel wedge support with cross-training (cycling). Sometimes a fasciotomy is necessary (Fig. 124).

Tibialis posterior dysfunction

This occurs in unfit middle-aged women as a result of degenerative changes in the tendon. The rupture may be partial or complete with pain (medial) and a flattened arch (a failed single stance heel raise test) (Fig. 125). Orthotic support, debridement or tendon transfer (of flexor digitorum longus) may be necessary.

Peroneal tendon subluxation/dislocation

This is seen in skiers (a violent ankle dorsiflexion in an avoidance manoeuvre) and a rim fracture (distal fibula) is apparent. Surgical reduction and stabilization is often necessary.

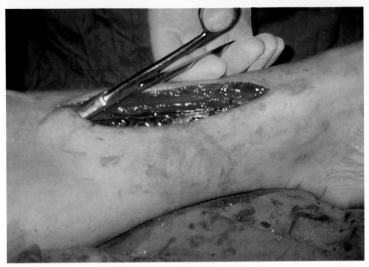

Fig. 124 Fasciotomy for compartment syndrome.

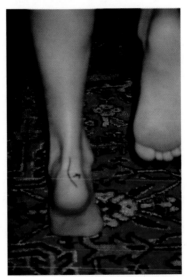

Fig. 125 Single stance heel raise test checks tibialis posterior function (positive where there is pain/weakness).

Tibiotalar spurs

Spurs of osteophytes may form on the lower anterior tibia or talar neck and cause impingement in dorsiflexion (Fig. 126). When significantly symptomatic, arthroscopic excision is indicated.

Os trigonum

This ossicle on the posterior aspect of the talus may cause pain with full plantar flexion (as in ballet pointing) (Fig. 127). It may be confused with flexor hallucis longus tendinitis. Should rest, NSAIDs and modification of activities fail, surgical excision is required.

Nerve entrapment

This is not uncommon about the foot and ankle but can be frustratingly difficult to treat.

Types   These include:

- anterior tarsal tunnel (the deep peroneal nerve under the inferior extensor retinaculum)
- tarsal tunnel (the tibial nerve compressed behind the medial malleolus) (Fig. 128)
- jogger's foot (the medial plantar nerve compressed at the knot of Henry)
- the sural nerve
- Morton's neuroma.

Treatment   Stretching, NSAIDs and orthotics may help, as may surgery where tenderness and symptoms can be anatomically localized.

Syndesmotic injuries

Syndesmotic or 'high' ankle sprains may be diagnosed by the squeeze test (Fig. 129) or the abduction/external rotation stress test. Casting for 4 weeks is required or surgical fixation where refractory.

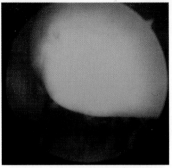

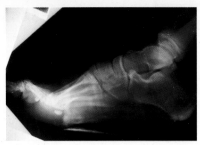

Fig. 127 Os trigonum.

Fig. 126 Tibiotalar spur at arthroscopy.

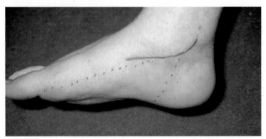

Fig. 128 Tarsal tunnel with area of decreased sensation.

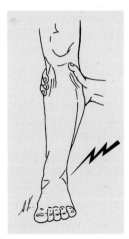

Fig. 129 Squeeze test positive for ankle pain from syndesmotic rupture.

12 / Injuries of the spine

The sight of a rugby player lying paralysed on a football field strikes fear into the hearts of relatives, coaches and spectators (Fig. 130).

Cervical (soft tissue) sprain

Mechanism of injury

A cervical sprain is caused by direct trauma, (collision) with an axial load and flexion (so-called 'whiplash' injury).

Clinical features

There is neck pain, stiffness and tension-type headache (occipital radiating to forehead).

X-rays and CT scans are normal. MRI is indicated if symptoms persist, especially where there are radicular symptoms.

Treatment

Treatment includes rest (initially), NSAIDs, soft collar (until spasm settles) and later physiotherapy. Exclude any neurological loss and ensure full range of motion of spine (before returning to sport) (Fig. 131).

Thoracic 'sprains'. In rowers, thoracic 'sprains' may be an exacerbation of their Scheuermann's disease.

Lumbar sprains. These are common. There is pain (often to the buttock), stiffness and loss of lumbar lordosis. Treatment consists of ice, NSAIDs, and sometimes a brace and back exercise programme.

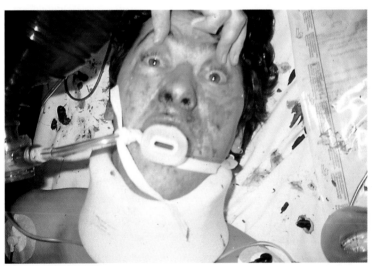

Highest
incidence

- Diving
- Snow mobile
- Equestrian
- Sky diving
- Football
- Skiing

Lowest incidence

- Mountaineering

Fig. 130 Sport and spinal injuries according to sport.

Fig. 131 Basal skull fracture with neck injury.

Fractures and dislocations

Cervical spine

Mechanism of injury
Fractures and dislocations of the cervical spine may be catastrophic. They result from axial loading (as in a dive or spear tackle). Boys with slender necks are probably more prone to injury.

On-field management—*cervical spine immobilization, airway control* and *safe transport*—is crucial (Fig. 132).

Clinical features
There may be neurological damage that is not fully apparent until the period of spinal shock is over (return of the bulbocavernosus reflex).

Treatment
Stable fractures require a cervical collar. Unstable fractures (>3.5 mm displacement or >20° angulation or neurological loss) require a halo-vest or surgical fixation. Intravenous steroids may be beneficial in the first 24 hours.

Facet dislocations (>25% displacement of one vertebral body on another is a unilateral facet dislocation; 50% displacement is bilateral) require reduction and stabilization. (A halo-vest or surgery is required for late instability.)

Neurological loss. This may be complete, i.e. quadriplegic (fracture at C3 is fatal as breathing is impossible because the phrenic nerve is from cranial nerves 4, 5 and 6), or incomplete (central, anterior, Brown-Sequard, posterior cord syndrome).

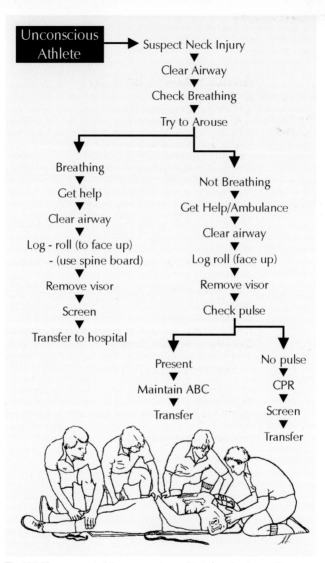

Unconscious Athlete → Suspect Neck Injury
▼
Clear Airway
▼
Check Breathing
▼
Try to Arouse

Breathing
▼
Get help
▼
Clear airway
▼
Log - roll (to face up)
- (use spine board)
▼
Remove visor
▼
Screen
▼
Transfer to hospital

Not Breathing
▼
Get Help/Ambulance
▼
Clear airway
▼
Log roll (face up)
▼
Remove visor
▼
Check pulse

Present
▼
Maintain ABC
▼
Transfer

No pulse
▼
CPR
▼
Screen
▼
Transfer

Fig. 132 Management of the unconscious athlete (caution here will prevent catastrophe).

Cervical spine (contd)

Particular injuries **C1 fracture (Jefferson).** A fracture of the ring of C1 seldom results in neurological loss and tends to be stable. It is often associated with cervical fractures. A halo-vest is required or later C1/2 surgical fusion.

Odontoid peg fracture (C2). A fracture may involve the tip (stable), base (unstable) or body (stable) of the peg. Exclude congenital abnormality (os odontoideum). A halo-vest is required but the base type is unstable and may need surgical stabilization (Fig. 133).

Hangman's fracture (C2). Pars fracture results from hyperextension. The fracture is stable and there is seldom neurological loss. A halo-vest is required and rarely surgery. Other cervical injuries should be excluded.

C3–7 fractures. These are compression fractures from an axial load (Figs 134, 135 & 136). Perform a neurological evaluation. A halo-vest is needed. Tear-drop fractures are stable. Unstable fractures require a halo-vest or surgical fixation.

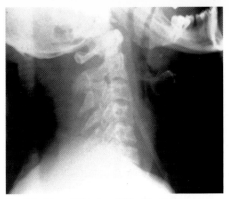

Fig. 133 Odontoid fracture (C1) with minimal displacement (check for second spinal injury).

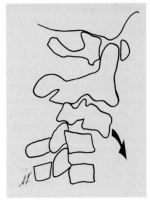

Fig. 134 C3/4 dislocation (>50% = both facets dislocated).

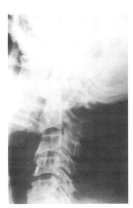

Fig. 135 C5 crush vertebral fracture.

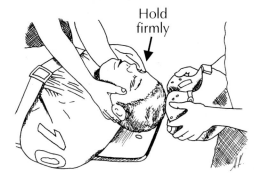

Hold firmly

Fig. 136 Remove helmet from patient (footballer) with assistant holding head.

Thoracic spine

Compression fractures. These usually involve the anterior column (exclude pathological fracture). Most are >25% (on lateral X-ray); where >50% there may be burst fragments in the canal (do a CT scan). Compression fractures are usually in the T10–L2 region (Fig. 137). Brace (6–12 weeks) in extension orthosis.

Fracture/dislocations. These are high-energy injuries with a high likelihood of spinal cord damage. Paraplegia may result (10% decrease in life expectancy).

Lumbar spine

Classification   Fractures of the lumbar spine are classified according to the three-column concept.

- *Posterior column fractures* (spinous/transverse process)—non-operative management.
- *Transverse process fractures* occur from powerful contraction of the psoas muscle (exclude renal damage) with paralytic ileus and loin haematoma.
- *Unstable fractures* (more than two columns) require surgical stabilization and no further contact sports.

Vertical ring apophysis injury. This is seen in wrestlers and female gymnasts. Disc material has pushed through the end plate. The injury is of doubtful significance.

Other cervical problems

Cervical stenosis. This is a congenital/developmental narrowing (anteroposterior; Fig. 138) and can predispose to neuropraxia (full recovery is the rule). It is probably safe to play sport. The condition is not uncommon with American football and skiing.

Cervical spine abnormalities. Where C1 and C2 are involved (e.g. Klipper–Feil), contact sport should be avoided.

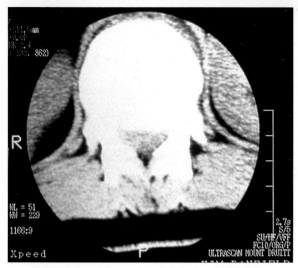

Fig. 137 T12 fracture with encroachment upon canal (CT picture of injured diver's spine).

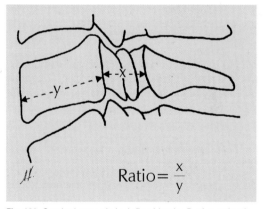

$$Ratio = \frac{x}{y}$$

Fig. 138 Cervical stenosis is defined by the Pavlov ratio x/y (<0.80).

Disc injury

Mechanism of injury
Injury usually occurs in the lumbar spine (L4/5, L5/ S1), sometimes the cervical spine (C4/5, C5/6, C6/7) and rarely the thoracic, as a result of bending or twisting.

Cervical disc rupture. This may result in transient quadriplegia (anterior cord syndrome—no motor/ sensory activity but intact sense of position/vibration). CT and MRI are useful.

Clinical features
Radiculopathy is seen (with loss of reflexes).

Treatment. Treatment includes analgesia, soft collar and gentle physiotherapy. Surgical partial disc excision and fusion may be required where severe symptoms persist.

After solid fusion (surgery), athletes may, if asymptomatic, return to contact sports, but not those with central disc herniations and 'hard' discs with neurological symptoms.

Lumbar disc rupture

Mechanism of injury
Lumbar disc rupture is not uncommon, especially in weight lifters. The disc desiccates, degenerates (with age) and bulges/extrudes/is sequestered (Fig. 139).

Clinical features
There is back pain with leg pain and nerve tension signs (nerve compression) (Fig. 140). Exclude a cauda equina problem (bowel/bladder dysfunction, saddle anaethesia and bilateral leg pain) as urgent surgery is then required.

Treatment
Treatment is rest, NSAIDs, traction, sometimes epidural steroids, and occasionally partial surgical excision. There is a definite recurrence rate after either conservative treatment or surgery of up to 20% (Fig. 141).

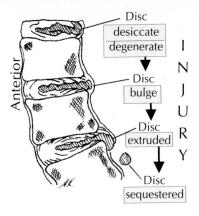

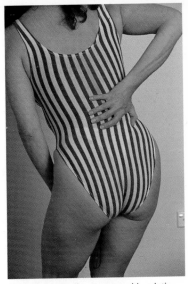

Fig. 139 Pathological sequence of disc disease leading to mechanical symptoms.

Fig. 140 Acute disc rupture with sciatic list and loss of lumber lordosis.

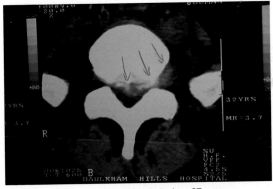

Fig. 141 Large disc herniation (extrusion) on CT scan.

Facet joint pain

Mechanism of injury
Injury is caused by rotation of the spine in tennis players and golfers. There is no leg pain.

Treatment
Rest, NSAIDs, physiotherapy and occasionally steroid facet injection.

Spear tackler's spine

Mechanism of injury
This is developmental cervical spine stenosis with loss of lordosis, and pre-existing radiographic abnormality. It occurs as a result of improper American football head collision tackling technique and head butting in rugby league (Fig. 142).

Clinical features
The condition presents as cervical spinal cord neuropraxia with transient quadriplegia (1 min to 48 h; resolves completely) or traumatic radiculopathy (burners and stingers).

Treatment
No further contact sports until the condition resolves.

Spondylolysis

Mechanism of injury
This is a stress fracture in the pars interarticularis, usually seen at the L5/S1 level. Fast bowlers in cricket, ballet dancers and gymnasts are prone to it.

Clinical features
Pain and stiffness are seen. An oblique X-ray best shows it (the 'Scottie dog' appearance) (Fig. 143).

Treatment
Symptomatic, rarely surgical fixation.
It is important to recognize the 'at risk' signs for progression to a slip (spondylolisthesis) (Fig. 144).

Spondylolisthesis

Mechanism of injury
This is a slip (anterior displacement of one vertebral body over another), usually at L4/5 level (and normally <25%). A slip at the L5/S1 level may progress to 100% displacement (spondyloptosis).

Clinical features
There is pain, stiffness and deformity (Fig. 145).

Treatment
Minor slips (<25%) require exercise and physiotherapy; severe slips surgical fusion.

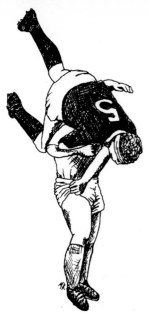

Fig. 142 Spear tackle in rugby.

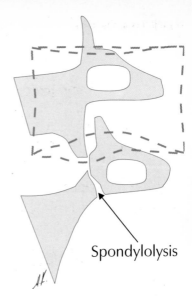

Spondylolysis

Fig. 143 'Scottie dog' appearance (with neck collar = pars defect) pathognomonic of spondylolysis.

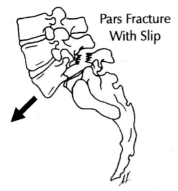

Pars Fracture With Slip

At risk for slip progression
- young age at presentation
- female
- high grade slip (>50%)
- dome shaped sacrum

Fig. 144 Spondylolisthesis (pars fracture with slip): risk factors.

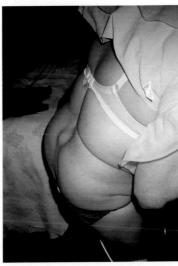

Fig. 145 Typical appearance of spondylolisthesis (heart-shaped buttocks, loin creases, palpable step off, flattening).

13 / **The child athlete**

To excel in sports today, the young athlete is forced to train longer, harder and start at an earlier age.

Child/adult differences

Children are not merely small adults. There are marked differences in coordination, strength and stamina. Children have lower anaerobic capabilities, are less metabolically efficient and have less efficient thermoregulatory mechanisms.

Their pattern of injury sustained differs significantly from that of the adult (Fig. 146). Adolescents sustain more injuries and more severe injuries than children (larger body mass and strength).

Musculoskeletal differences

Effects of growth/ immature skeleton

The effects of growth and the special properties of the immature skeleton that affect the type of injury sustained by children (Figs 147 & 148) are:

- Children's bone is plastic (hence bow deformity as a result of plastic deformation of long bones is seen in children; greenstick and torus fractures occur).
- Ligament and tendon injuries are less frequent than epiphyseal and apophyseal injuries (the joint capsule and ligament in a child is two to five times stronger than the epiphyseal plate).
- The growth cartilage is susceptible to stress. Children are therefore more susceptible to overuse injuries.
- Mismatch between bone and soft tissue growth during the adolescent growth spurt causes muscle–tendon tightness, loss of flexibility and increased risk of overuse injuries.

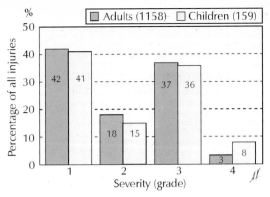

Fig. 146 Overall children skiing injuries tend to be more severe (Snowy Mountains, 1984).

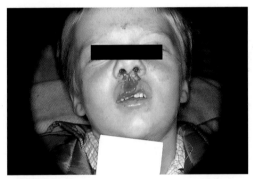

Fig. 147 Facial injury in young skier.

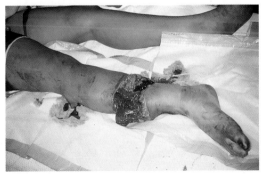

Fig. 148 Open fibial fracture with major nerve and vessel injury requiring immediate amputation.

Macrotrauma

Children are injured from a single impact (macrotrauma) or repetitive overuse injury (microtrauma).

Bone injuries occur more readily than ligamentous injuries (intraligementous injuries and muscle tears are rare). X-ray examinations are always indicated in sprains and strains to exclude bone, epiphyseal or apophyseal injuries.

Common injuries

The more common injuries include fractures of the wrist, radius, ulna, clavicle, tibia and fibula, and dislocations of the shoulder, elbow and interphalangeal joints of the hand (Fig. 149).

Of special note in children

Valgus and varus stress injuries to the knee. These may present as joint laxity. (The laxity will show as a fracture of the growth plate of the distal femur/proximal tibia on stress X-ray.) Distal femoral physeal injury has a higher incidence of growth discrepancy than physeal injury elsewhere (Fig. 150).

Distal fibular epiphyseal injury. An injury of the distal fibular epiphysis (growth plate injury) presents as a lateral ligament injury (do not confuse with normal accessory ossification centres at the fibular tip).

Tibial spine fracture. This is an epiphyseal injury (Fig. 151) (equivalent of an isolated adult anterior cruciate ligament tear). Instability may result.

Acute traumatic separation of the upper femoral epiphysis (SUFE). True acute SUFE is rare (acute exacerbation of chronic epiphyseal slip is not infrequent). Complications include malunion and dreaded avascular necrosis.

Meniscal injury. This is uncommon. A *discoid meniscus* produces a 'clicking sensation' and/or lateral pain.

Ligament injuries. Anterior cruciate and collateral ligament injuries can occur (especially in adolescents). Surgery is required when there is instability.

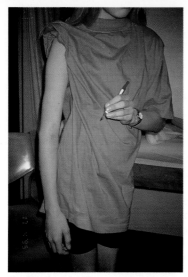

Fig. 149 Brachial plexus paralysis from trampoline injury.

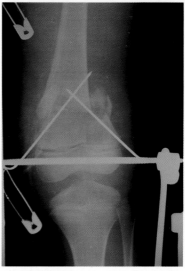

Fig. 150 Distal femoral growth plate injury (reduced/held with wires/traction).

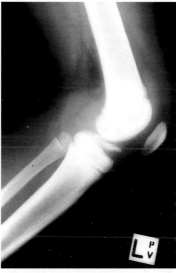

Fig. 151 Displaced tibial spine fracture.

Of special note in children (contd)

Avulsion

- Avulsion of the tibial tubercle may occur when landing with a flexed knee (or become symptomatic from chronic overuse) (Fig. 152). It occurs in boys (14–16 years).
- Acute avulsion of the anterior superior iliac spine, anterior inferior iliac spine, ischial apophysis or, more rarely, iliac apophysis and lesser trochanter occur with sudden overload of the muscle tendon unit that inserts on the apophysis (the sartorius, rectus femoris, hamstring, abdominal muscles and iliopsoas).

Injuries of the head and neck

Injuries of the head and neck have serious social and economic impact.

Spinal cord injuries

Incidence Child athletes are less susceptible to spinal cord injuries (Fig. 153), possibly due to the intrinsic properties of the immature spine, smaller weight or less speed. Most occur from diving accidents, gymnastics and rugby. Most involve the cervical spine and more often (than motor vehicle accidents) produce quadriplegia. Up to 80% of diving injuries to the cervical spine result in quadriplegia.

Mechanism of injury There may be an obvious fracture (especially in children under 11 years). Axial loading of the slightly flexed neck is the mechanism (striking the head on the bottom in a diving accident, head butting, spear tackling, scrum collapse in rugby and American football (Fig. 154). Most neck injuries in gymnastics occur on the trampoline.

Prevention Rules and equipment changes reduce the incidence of serious spinal injuries. (Perhaps matching teams for weight and skill, rather than age alone.)

Head injuries. These occur in cycling and boxing (Fig. 155). (Serious head injury is uncommon in youth boxing but the incidence of chronic brain injury is not known.)

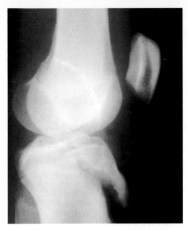

Fig. 152 Avulsed tibial tubercle from leap in basketball.

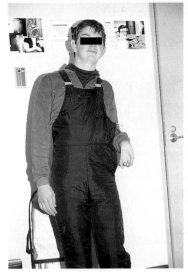

Fig. 153 Boy with left hemiparesis and frontal lesion (motor vehicle accident) but still able and keen to ski.

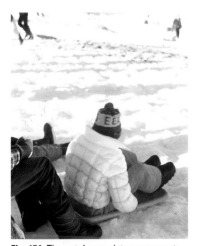

Fig. 154 These tobogganists are prone to spinal injuries.

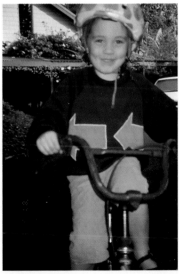

Fig. 155 Head injuries are prevented by proper use of helmets.

Microtrauma (overuse injuries)

Children are more prone to injury from repetitive compression, tension, torsion or shear stresses on bone, ligaments, tendons or cartilage at junctional areas.

Sports-specific injuries

- Overhead throwing sports (baseball) cause repetitive traction on the medial side of the elbow and compression on the lateral side (little league elbow), producing overgrowth of the medial epicondyle, medial soft tissue tears, osteochondritis dissecans of the capitellum and radial head, fatigue of the proximal humeral physis (Figs 156 & 157).
- More than 50% of champion swimmers suffer shoulder pain ('swimmer's shoulder') from impingement, laxity and overuse (Fig. 158).
- Young female gymnasts have a four times higher risk of stress fractures of the pars interarticularis.

Overuse injuries unique to the child athlete include osteochondroses and stress fractures.

Osteochondroses

Definition

These are a broad group of conditions with similar radiological features from focal disturbances of the endochondrial ossification. They may be avascular in origin (Kienböck's disease) or result from mechanical stresses on susceptible epiphyses or apophyses (differentiate from ossification variants).

Types

There are three types of osteochondrosis: articular, non-articular and physeal.

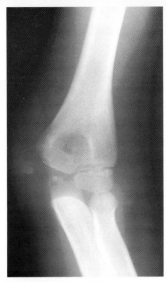

Fig. 156 Medial condylar fracture from basketball.

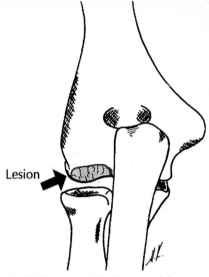

Fig. 157 Osteochondritis dissecans of the capitellum (Panner's disease).

Lesion

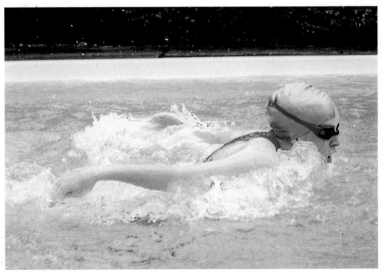

Fig. 158 Swimmers (especially with butterfly stroke) are prone to impingement problems.

Articular osteochondrosis

Definition This is a localized area of subchondral demarcation, with or without involvement of the overlying articular cartilage.

Cause The cause is uncertain (genetic, trauma, ischaemia or separation of an abnormal ossification). It is seen in the hip (Perthes' disease), the lower femur (knee; Fig. 159), patella, talus, navicular (Kohler's disease), metatarsal (Freiberg's disease; Fig. 160), lower humerus (Panner's disease), radial head, lunate (Kienböck's disease).

Non-articular osteochondrosis

Types *Osgood–Schlatter's disease.* This is caused by fatigue avulsion of a portion of the immature tibial tubercle (Fig. 161). It is common in athletic children (boys at 13 years).

Sinding-Larsen–Johansson disease. This is a stress avulsion injury at the lower (and sometimes upper) pole of the patella. The condition is self-limiting but may require cessation of activities (up to 3 months cylinder cast immobilization helps).

Physeal osteochondrosis

Scheuermann's disease is a cause of juvenile onset throacic kyphosis. Anterior vertebral wedging, end plate irregularities and Schmorl's nodes formation are seen on X-ray examination (Fig. 162). The aetiology is unknown.

Treatment Dorsal kyphosis of less than 50° is rarely symptomatic and requires no active treatment. (Brace treatment is required for symptomatic kyphosis of more than 50°.) Surgery is seldom required. Neurological complications are rare (usually associated with trauma).

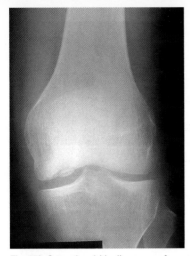

Fig. 159 Osteochondritis dissecans of medial femoral condyle (usual site) knee.

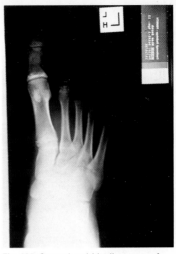

Fig. 160 Osteochondritis dissecans of head of second metatarsal (Freiberg's disease).

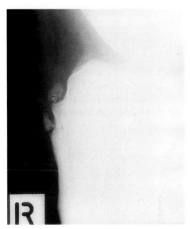

Fig. 161 Osgood–Schlatter's disease.

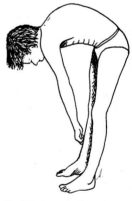

Fig. 162 Juvenile thoracic kyphosis (Scheuermann's disease) is accentuated on forward flexion.

Stress fractures

Incidence The incidence and pattern of stress fractures differ in children (less than 10% occur under 15 years old). The tibia is the most common site at all ages (50% of all), followed by metatarsals, fibula, femur and vertebra (pars) (Figs 163 & 164).

Types Stress fractures are either:

- *fatigue-type* (abnormal stress on normal bone), or
- *insufficiency-type* (normal stress on deficient bone) and can occur as a result of muscular stress on bone.

Mechanism of injury Fracture occurs after new, strenuous and repetitive activities (following inactivity). A small cortical crack starts and propagates by subcortical infarction.

Location The usual site is at the junction of the metaphysis and diaphysis. Some are sports-specific (pars interarticularis fractures from chronic hyperextension of the lumbar spine in competitive gymnasts and cricket bowlers).

Clinical features There may be systemic symptoms of listlessness and even pyrexia. Osteoid osteoma, subacute osteomyelitis, Ewing's sarcoma and osteogenic sarcoma *must* be differentiated from stress fractures (Fig. 165).

X-ray examination will identify 50% of stress fractures. A positive bone scan may be expected for almost all cases.

Prevention Stress fractures can be prevented by proper conditioning and intelligent introduction of new training regimes.

Treatment Treatment is by rest and graduated return to sports. Stress fractures of the tibia may be recalcitrant and persist for many months. (Difficult cases may require electrical stimulation.)

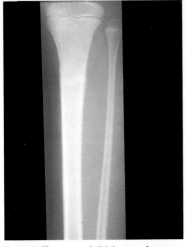

Fig. 163 (Transverse) tibial stress fracture seen only on bone scan.

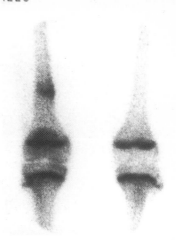

Fig. 164 Femoral stress fracture seen only on bone scan.

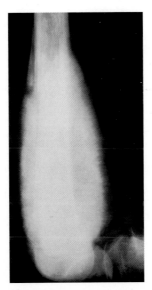

Fig. 165 High grade osteogenic sarcoma of the femur (X-rays are important).

14 / **The older athlete**

Definition The older athlete may be:

- anyone older than the current world record holder for a particular event.
- anyone considered 'old' in the community, or
- anyone older than yourself.

Inactivity This accounts for more than half the physiological and structural decline in sedentary adults. Warm-up and warm-down periods with exercise are important.

Changes with ageing

Musculoskeletal system

Collagen and elastin. Increased molecular stability and brittleness of structures means less compliance and therefore vulnerability to disruption.

Tendon and ligament. These are also less compliant with reduced glycosaminoglycan content. Bone resorption at tendon or ligament insertion occurs, with less force required to avulse them.

Skeletal muscle. There is loss of muscle mass (5–10%) by reduction in the number and size of fibres. Fast twitch (type II) are lost more than slow twitch (type I). However, metabolic capacity remains fairly stable. Strength falls slowly until about 50 years old; thereafter there is a more rapid decline—approximately 10–20% by age 60. Power (= work/time) is reduced because of slower muscle contraction.

Bone. Loss of bone mass occurs normally with ageing after the third or fourth decade, due to reduction in osteoblastic activity. This is accelerated in women after the menopause. Trabecular bone is more affected than cortical bone (Figs 166 & 167).

Cartilage. Water content is reduced; smaller proteoglycan subunits result in less ability to withstand compression and deformation. However, inactivity is the greatest accelerator of cartilage deterioration (Fig. 168, p. 118).

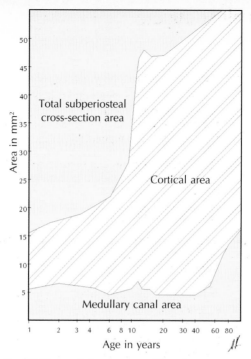

Fig. 166 Changes in bone contour with ageing.

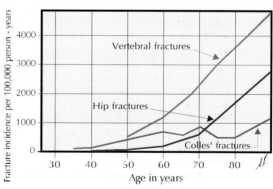

Fig. 167 Fracture pattern with ageing.

Cardiovascular system
The maximum cardiac workload reduces with age. This may be accelerated by atherosclerosis. The ageing heart has to work harder to meet the same metabolic demands (Fig. 169).

Respiratory system
Functional lung reserves for aerobic work efforts are reduced and so also the respiratory system's ability to deliver oxygen to the body's working cellular systems.

Central nervous system
Athletic performance is affected by decreases in:

- fluid (new and complex task) intelligence
- attention spans
- reaction times.

Temperature regulation
Older athletes are more prone to heat accumulation (heat exhaustion) and heat loss (hypothermia).

Musculoskeletal risk areas for older athletes

Older athletes are more prone to:

- rotator cuff and bicipital tendinitis (Fig. 170)
- patellofemoral arthrosis
- trochanteric (hip) bursitis
- quadriceps tendinitis and rupture
- gastrocnemius tear
- osteoporotic fractures (in postmenopausal women)
- discogenic low back pain.

Psychosocial benefits of exercise

Athletic participation has innumerable benefits for older athletes in terms of continuing to participate in society. They suffer less tension, fatigue, depression, confusion and anger, and have improved vigour (Fig. 171).

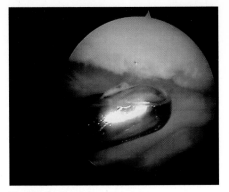

Fig. 168 Cartilage damage in knee (arthroscopic chondroplasty).

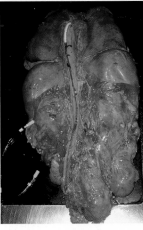

Fig. 169 Balloon pump (in situ at autopsy) has failed to maintain cardiac output.

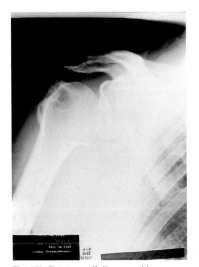

Fig. 170 Rotator cuff disease with osteophytes.

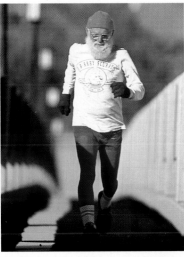

Fig. 171 Exercise delays physical decline.

Index

Abdominal injuries, 19
Achilles tendon injuries, 83, 84
Acromioclavicular joint injuries, 35, 36
Adductor strain, 61
Ageing, 115–117
Altitude medicine, 9–10
Amenorrhoea, exercise-associated, 23–24
Amphetamines, 21
Anabolic steroids, 21, 22
Anaemia, 29
Ankle
    Achilles tendon injuries, 83, 84
    fractures, 81, 82
    impingement, 29
    nerve entrapment, 89
    sprains/instability, 79–80
    stress fractures, 85
    syndesmotic injuries, 89, 90
Ankylosis, elbow, 48
Anorexia nervosa, 27
Anterior cruciate ligament tears, 73, 74
    children, 105
    female athletes, 29
Anterior talofibular ligament (ATFL), tears,
    79, 80

Barotrauma (BT), 13–14
Baseball finger see Mallet finger
Bennett's fracture, 51
Biceps
    distal biceps rupture, 47
    rupture of long head, 39, 40
    tendinitis, 39
Blood doping, 21
Boutonnière deformity, 53, 54
Brachial plexus palsy, 39, 106
Bulimia nervosa, 27
Bunions, 29
Bursitis, pelvic area, 61, 62

Calcaneofibular ligament, tears, 79, 80
Calcaneus, fracture, 81
Cardiac death, sudden, 15, 21
Cardiovascular function, 3
Carpal tunnel syndrome, 49, 50
Cerebral oedema, altitude, 9
Charley horse, 59
Chest injuries, 19
Child athlete
    head and neck injuries, 107–108
    injury pattern, 103, 104
    lower limb injuries, 105–107, 108
    musculoskeletal differences, 103
    osteochondroses, 109–112
    overuse injuries, 109–114
    stress fractures, 113–114
Chondromalacia patellae, 75, 76
Chronic fatigue syndrome, 21

Clavicle, outer, osteolysis, 37
Cold stress, 7–9
Collateral ligaments of knee, tears, 73, 74
    children, 106
Compartment syndrome, 87, 88
Computerized tomography (CT), head
    injuries, 17, 18
Contraception, 29
Corked thigh, 59
Cruciate ligament, anterior see Anterior
    cruciate ligament
Cubital tunnel nerve compression
    syndrome, 47

Death, sudden, 15–20, 21
Decompression sickness (DCS), 11
Dental injuries, 17, 20
Disabled athletes, 21, 22
Diving, underwater, 11–14
    causes of death, 12
Drug abuse, 21
Dupuytren's fracture, 81

Eating disorders, 27–28
Elbow, valgus stress testing, 43, 44
Elbow injuries, 41–48
    children, 109, 110
    dislocation, 43, 44
    fractures, 43, 110
    loose bodies, 45, 46
    nerves, 45, 46, 47, 48
    valgus extension overload, 43, 44
Endurance training, 1
Environment, 5–14
Epiphysis, medial humeral, separation from
    distal humerus, 41, 42
Exercise, 1–3
    capacity, 3
    types, 3
Exercise-associated amenorrhoea (EAA),
    23–24

Faciomaxillary injuries, 17, 20
Fasciotomy, compartment syndrome, 87, 88
Fatigue, 1
    chronic fatigue syndrome, 21
Female athletes, 23–30
Femur
    fractured femur and pelvis, 69, 70
    growth plate injury, 105, 106
    osteogenic sarcoma, 114
    slip of upper femoral epiphysis (SUFE),
        67, 68, 105
    stress fractures, 67, 68, 114
Fibular epiphyseal injury, distal, 105
Finger injuries, 53–56
Flexor digitorum profundus tendon
    avulsion, 53, 54

Foot
   female athlete, 29
   fractures, 81, 82
   nerve entrapment, 89, 90
   osteochondritis dissecans, 112
   stress fractures, 85
Freiberg's disease, 111, 112

Gamekeeper's thumb, 55, 56
Glandular fever, 21
Golfer's elbow, 43
Groin strain, 61
Growth hormone, 21
Growth plate injury, 105, 106
Guyon's canal syndrome, 49

Haematomas, intracranial, 17
Hamate, hook of hamate fracture, 51, 52
Hammer toes, 29
Hamstrings
   strains, 63, 64
   stretching, 4
Hand injuries, 49–56
   fingers/thumb, 53–56
   nerves, 50, 51
   tendinitis, 50, 51
Handlebar palsy, 49
Hangman's fracture, 95
Head injuries, 17–18, 20
   children, 107, 108
Heat illnesses, 5–6
Heel raise test, single stance, 87, 88
Hepatitis, 21
Hip injuries, 59, 60, 61
   conjoint tendon strain, 64, 65
   dislocation, 67, 68
   fractures, 67, 68
   hip joint strain, 64, 65
   irritable hip, 64
   labral tears, 65, 66
   osteoarthritis, 69, 70
   snapping hip, 64
Hip pointer, 61
HIV infection, 21
Human growth hormone, 21
Hyperthermia, 5–6
   and sudden death, 15
Hypothermia, 7–9
   and sudden death, 15

Iliac crest
   apophysitis and avulsion, 63
   contusion, 61
Iliac spines, avulsion, 59, 60
Ilio-inguinal nerve entrapment, 65, 66
Iliotibial band friction syndrome, 77, 78
Interosseous nerves, compression, 47
Interphalangeal joint injuries, hand, 53–56
Intersection syndrome, 49, 50
Intervertebral disk injury, 99–100
Iron deficiency, 29
Ischial apophysitis (bursitis) and avulsion,
   61, 62

Jefferson fracture, 95

Jersey finger see Flexor digitorum profundus
   tendon avulsion
Jogger's foot, 89
Jumper's knee, 77, 78

Kienböîck's disease, 109, 110
Knee injuries, 71–78
   cartilage damage, older athlete, 118
   children, 105–106
   ligaments, 73–74, 106
   meniscal tears, 71–72, 105
   osteochondritis dissecans, 111, 112
   patellofemoral joint, 29, 75–77, 78
   plicas, 77, 78
Kohler's disease, 111
Kyphosis, juvenile-onset thoracic, 111, 112

Labral tears
   hip, 65, 66
   shoulder, 37, 38
Lachman's test, 73, 74
Lactic acid, 1
Lateral collateral ligament tears (LCL) of
   knee, tears, 73
Leg injuries, 85–90
   children, 105–107, 108, 111–112
   see also Thigh
Little league elbow, 41, 42, 109
Lunotriquetral ligament tears, 57, 58

Maisonneuve fracture, 81, 82
Mallet finger, 53, 54
Mandible, fracture, 17, 20
Maxilla, fracture, 17, 20
Medial collateral ligament (MCL) of knee,
   tears, 73, 74
Median nerve compression, wrist, 49
Menarche, delayed, 23
Meniscal tears, knee, 71–72
Menstrual disorders, 23–24
Menstruation, effect on performance, 29, 30
Metabolism, anaerobic/aerobic, 1
Muscle action, 1, 2
Muscle fibres, 1
Metacarpals, fractures, 51
Metacarpophalangeal (MCP) dislocations,
   55, 56
Morton's neuroma, 89
Mountain sickness, 9
Muscle ruptures, shoulder, 39, 40
Musculoskeletal injuries, females, 29, 30
Myositis ossificans traumatica, thigh, 9, 60

Navicular fractures, 81
Neck
   abnormalities, 97
   crush fracture, 16
   disc injury, 99
   fractures/dislocations, 93–96
   injuries, children, 107, 108
   sprain, 91
   stenosis, 97
Necrosis, avascular, 69, 70

Obturator nerve entrapment, 65, 66

O'Donoghue's unhappy triad, 73
Odontoid peg fracture, 95, 96
Older athlete
  benefits of exercise, 118
  changes with ageing, 115–117
  risk areas, 117
Oligomenorrhoea, 23, 24
Os trigonum, 89, 90
Osgood-Schlatter's disease, 77, 111, 112
Osteitis pubic, 65
Osteochondritis dissecans
  elbow, 41, 42, 45, 109, 110
  lower limb, children, 111, 112
Osteochondrosis, 109
  articular, 111
  non-articular, 111
  physeal, 111
Osteolysis, outer clavicular, 37
Osteoporosis, 25, 26
Osteorathritis, elbow, 45, 46, 48

Panner's disease, 41, 42, 110, 111
Paronychia, 29
Patella
  alta/baja, 77
  chondromalacia, 75, 76
  dislocated, 76
  lateral patellar compression syndrome, 75
  maltracking, 75, 76
  tenditis, 77, 78, 111
Patellofemoral joint injuries, 29, 75–77, 78
Pectoralis major, rupture, 39
Pelvic injuries, 61, 62
  fracture, 69, 70
Peroneal tendon subluxation/dislocation, 87
Perthes' disease, 111
Phalanges, fractures, 51
Plantar fasciitis, 83
Pneumothorax, 19, 20
Pregnancy, 29
Pronator syndrome, 47
Psychology, 3
Pubic symphysitis, 65
Pulmonary function, 3
Pulmonary oedema, altitude, 9

Quadriceps femoris injuries, 59, 60

Radius, distal fracture, 51, 52
Respiratory tract, upper, infections of, 21
Resuscitation, 19
Retinal haemorrhage, at altitude, 9
Rotator cuff
  disease, with osteophytes, 118
  tears, 35, 36
  tendinitis, 29, 30

Sarcoma, osteogenic, of femur, 114
Scaphoid fracture, 51, 52, 58
Scapholunate ligament tears, 57, 58
Scheuermann's disease, 111, 112
Shoulder
  dislocation, 31–34
  impingement, 35, 36, 109, 110
  instability, 31–34, 36, 39

muscle ruptures, 39, 40
nerve injuries, 39, 40
subluxation, 31, 33, 34, 36
swimmer's, 109, 110
tendinitis, 35
Simmond's test, 83, 84
Sinding-Larsen-Johansson syndrome (SLJ), 77, 78, 111
Skier's hip, 67
Skier's thumb, 55, 56
Spear tackler's spine, 101, 102
Spine, 92
  cervical, abnormalities, 97
  cervical (soft tissue) sprain, 91–92
  cervical stenosis, 97, 98, 101
  child athlete, 107, 108
  disc injury, 99–100
  facet joint pain, 101
  female athlete, 29
  fractures/dislocations, 93–97, 98, 107
  spear tackler's, 101, 102
  spondylosis/spondylolisthesis, 29, 101, 102
Spondylolisthesis, 101, 102
Spondylolysis, 29, 101, 102
Spondyloptosis, 101
Sprint training, 1
'Squeakers' see Intersection syndrome
Sternoclavicular dislocation, 37, 38
Steroids, anabolic, 21, 22
Stress fractures
  children, 113–114
  femur, 67, 68
  lower limb, 85–86, 114
  spine, 101, 102
  women, 25
Stretching, 3, 4
Subscapularis muscle, rupture, 39
Sural nerve, entrapment, 89
'Swimmer's shoulder', 109, 110

Talofibular ligament, anterior, tears, 79, 80
Talus, fracture, 81, 82
Tarsal tunnel, 89
  anterior, 89
Tarsometatarsal fractures, 81, 82
Temperature extremes, 5–8
Tendinitis
  Achilles tendon, 83, 84
  biceps, 39
  de Quervain's, 49, 50
  hand and wrist, 50, 51
  patella, 77, 78
  shoulder, 29, 30, 35
Tennis elbow, 42, 43
Tennis leg, 83
Terry Thomas sign, 57
Thigh
  avascular necrosis, 69, 70
  fractures, 69–69
  muscle injuries, 59, 60
  nerve injuries, 65, 66
Thoracic nerve, long, injury to, 39, 40
Thumb, skier's (gamekeeper's), 55, 56
Tibia, stress fractures, 114
Tibial spine fracture, 105, 106

Tibial tubercle, avulsion, 107, 108
Tibialis posterior dysfunction, 87
Tibiotalar spurs, 89, 90
Training, 1
Traumatic deaths, 15
Triangular fibrocartilage complex (TFCC) tears, 57, 58
Triceps, distal triceps rupture, 47, 48
Trochanteric bursitis, 61, 62
Turf toe, 83, 84

Ulnar collateral ligament injuries, 43
Ulnar nerve injuries, 45, 46, 49
Underwater medicine, 11–14

Upper respiratory tract infections, 21

Vaginitis, 29
Vertebral body apophysitis, 29, 30

Watson's tests, 57
Weaver's bottom *see* Ischial apophysitis and avulsion
'Whiplash' injury, 91
Women, 23–30
Wrist injuries, 49–58
    fractures, 51–52
    nerves, 50, 51
    tendinitis, 50, 51